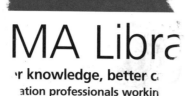

Clinical Hypertension

SECOND EDITION

in Practice

Sern Lim

University Department of Medicine, City
Hospital NHS Trust, Birmingham, UK

2003 First edition
2007 Second edition
Published by the Royal Society of Medicine Press Ltd
1 Wimpole Street, London W1G 0AE, UK
Tel: +44 (0) 20 7290 2921
Fax: +44 (0) 20 7290 2929
Email: publishing@rsm.ac.uk
Website: www.rsmpress.co.uk

The authors are responsible for the scientific content and for the views expressed, which are not necessarily those of the Royal Society of Medicine or of the Royal Society of Medicine Press Ltd.

Although every effort has been made to ensure that, where provided, information concerning drug dosages or product usage has been presented accurately in this publication, the ultimate responsibility rests with the prescribing physician and neither the publisher nor the sponsor can be held responsible for errors or any consequences arising from the use of information contained herein.

British Library Cataloguing in Publication Data

A catalogue record for this book is available from the British Library

ISBN 1-85315-659-0
ISSN 1473 6845

Distribution in Europe and Rest of World:
Marston Book Services Ltd
PO Box 269
Abingdon
Oxon OX14 4YN, UK
Tel: +44 (0) 1235 465 500
Fax: +44 (0) 1235 465 555
Email: direct.order@marston.com

Distribution in Australia and New Zealand:
Elsevier Australia
30–52 Smidmore Street
Marrickville NSW 2204
Australia
Tel: + 61 2 9517 8999
Fax: + 61 2 9517 2249
Email: service@elsevier.com.au

Distribution in the USA and Canada:
Royal Society of Medicine Press Ltd
c/o BookMasters, Inc
30 Amberwood Parkway
Ashland, Ohio 44805, USA
Tel: +1 800 247 6553 / +1 800 266 5564
Fax: +1 419 281 6883
E-mail: order@bookmasters.com

Typeset by Phoenix Photosetting, Chatham, Kent
Printed and bound in Spain by Liberdúplex

Foreword

The guidelines for the management of hypertension have progressively redefined this condition over the last few decades. Systemic hypertension, as it is now defined, encompasses a larger proportion of the population, but its significance as a cardiovascular risk factor is by no means diminished. Indeed, hypertension remains the major risk factor for cardiovascular morbidity and mortality. It is perhaps not surprising, therefore, that some of the largest clinical studies in recent years have been devoted to the management of high blood pressure. The data from these studies have prompted the release of new practice guidelines by the British Hypertension Society, the Joint British Societies and a further update by the National Institute for Health and Clinical Excellence.

This second edition of *Clinical Hypertension in Practice* builds on the strengths of the previous edition, with a new, young, dynamic author. The succinct description of the epidemiology, pathophysiology and clinical management of patients with hypertension is complemented by a clear summary of contemporary practice guidelines. This second edition should be of clear value to general practitioners, hospital doctors, students and nurses.

Gregory YH Lip

Professor of Cardiovascular Medicine
University Department of Medicine
City Hospital, Birmingham
UK

About the author

Hoong Sern Lim MD MRCP (London) is a Specialist Registrar in Cardiology at the West Midlands Deanery, UK. He has interests in clinical (diabetes, hypertension and heart failure) and basic science research (vascular biology), and has published numerous times on these subjects. He is a member of the European Society of Cardiology's Working Group on Pathogenesis of Atherosclerosis.

Preface

Interest in the arterial pulse and blood pressure date back hundreds, if not thousands of years. However, it was not until the pioneering work of Hales in 1733 and the description of stethoscopic sounds by Korotkoff in 1905 (and no less significant contributions of many others in the intervening years) that blood pressure measurement became established. These pioneering works thus allowed the study of the arterial blood pressure to grow from anecdotal to objective. Epidemiological studies that followed only a few decades later established high blood pressure as a major risk factor for cardiovascular disease.

Hamilton, Thompson and Wisniewski first published a clinical trial on the treatment of high blood pressure in 1964. This study signalled the beginning of an era of large placebo-controlled trials in the treatment of hypertension, which coincided with the development of new antihypertensive therapy, most notably the calcium channel blockers, angiotensin-converting enzyme inhibitors and angiotensin II receptor blockers. These clinical trials have shaped, and continue to shape, contemporary clinical guidelines. Indeed, the British Hypertension Society guidelines for the management of hypertension have undergone several revisions since Swales chaired the working party that prepared the Society's first report in 1989.

This book provides an overview of the historical, pathophysiological and clinical aspects of hypertension. The chapters on the diagnosis and management (both pharmacological and non-pharmacological) incorporate the British Hypertension Society (2004) and the Joint British Societies (2005) guidelines, and the most recent guidance update by the National Institute for Health and Clinical Excellence (NICE) and British Hypertension Society in 2006.

Sern Lim
September 2006

Contents

1. Historical background

The description of a 'hard pulse disease' dates back as far back as 2600 BC. In 1555, Joseph Struthius first described a primitive method of quantifying blood pressure by determining the number of objects that have to be placed to suppress the arterial pulsation. However, it was not until the series of experiments by Stephen Hales in the early 1700s that the basis of blood pressure measurement became established. Hales measured pressure in the leg and neck vessels of various animals and meticulously documented his observations. For example:

> 'In the larger horse and ox, the blood pressure is higher and the pulse slower than in the smaller sheep and dog'
> 'With blood loss, the pulse quickens and weakens and the blood pressure falls'
> 'Horses died when the blood pressure fell below 2 feet of blood'
> 'Blood pressure is increased during systole'

In the 1830s, with only a candle, a spoon, some acid (to distinguish phosphate from albumin) and pioneering clinical-pathological studies, Richard Bright was able to demonstrate the link between albuminuria, a hardened pulse and hypertrophy of the heart, particularly affecting the left ventricle. However, he had no means to quantify the blood pressure. This link between blood pressure and 'Bright's disease' (nephritis) was only described later by Frederick Mohamed in the 1870s with his modified sphygmograph. With his sphygmograph, Mohamed was able to document the presence of 'morbid arterial tension' in the absence of albuminuria. He called this 'chronic Bright's disease without albuminuria', now more familiar to us as essential hypertension. Mohamed also noted changes in the pulse waveform in persons with elevated arterial pressure and the elderly ('the tidal wave is prolonged and too much sustained'), which formed the basis of 'premature arterial senility'.

During this period, William Gull and Henry Sutton (in 1872) described the pathological changes in the kidneys in advanced stages of Bright's disease. They called the lesions 'arterio-capillary fibrosis', corresponding to arteriosclerosis of today. They also noted the presence of these lesions in other organs, including the heart, which was always hypertrophied. Gull and Sutton considered the arterio-capillary fibrosis an affection of the whole arterial system. Hence, the clinical and pathological changes in hypertensive disease were recognized by the end of the 19th century, and the study of arterial blood pressure was ready for the transition from the anecdotal to the objective.

The early years of the 20th century witnessed the introduction of the cuff sphygmomanometer and the seminal work by Nikolai Korotkoff. In 1905, Korotkoff presented his new method of measuring blood pressure at a scientific seminar of the Imperial Military Medical Academy in St Petersburg, Russia. In his studies, Korotkoff used Riva-Rocci's technique, first proposed in 1896, which involved an arm-encircling inflatable elastic cuff, a rubber bulb to inflate the cuff and a mercury sphygmomanometer. Riva-Rocci used this apparatus to measure systolic blood pressure by palpating the radial pulse. In 1897, Hill and Barnard reported a similar arm-encircling inflatable cuff apparatus to measure systolic blood pressure using a needle pressure gauge instead of palpation. Korotkoff's method, however, was a significant improvement over these other two techniques as it allowed measurement of diastolic blood pressure and, with the auscultatory technique, offered greater accuracy. Indeed, systolic blood pressure by Korotkoff's techniques was consistently 10–12 mmHg higher than the palpation method because generation of the pulse required filling of the vessel.

Korotkoff's contribution proved to be the catalyst in hypertension research. His method was widely received and quickly became a standard medical procedure. By 1916, data had been presented to show the relationship between risk of death and systolic blood pressure in asymptomatic individuals. Numerous epidemiological studies followed, clearly documenting the risk of high blood pressure.

At the same time, the treatment of hypertension developed apace. Early use of sodium thiocyanate and sympathectomy in the early 20th century to treat high blood pressure was unsurprisingly unpopular. The first major breakthrough came serendipitously when researchers working with the antibiotic sulphanilamide noted increased diuresis in their patients, which led to the development of chlorothiazide in the 1950s. Also in the 1950s and '60s, Sir James Black, building upon the work by Raymond Ahlquist in 1948 on adrenergic receptors, pioneered research into pharmacological intervention of the adrenergic system, which culminated in the development of beta-blockers. The first beta-blocker, propranolol, was introduced in 1964. The development of angiotensin-converting enzyme (ACE) inhibitors also started in the 1960s when an ACE inhibitor prototype was isolated from the Brazilian pit viper venom. In 1975, Cushman and Ondetti manipulated the carboxypeptidase A inhibitor and produced the first synthetic inhibitor of ACE, captopril.

By the middle part of the 20th century, the growing epidemiological data on the hazards of high blood pressure and emergence of (then untested) therapeutic agents set the scene for clinical trials for the treatment of asymptomatic patients with hypertension. In 1958, Hamilton and colleagues started the recruitment of patients for the first controlled trial with ganglion-blocking drugs (later replaced with methyldopa) and thiazide diuretics. Their landmark study of 61 patients was published in 1964 and demonstrated the benefit of blood pressure treatment. It was followed by a series of (much larger) studies, which have shaped contemporary guidelines for the treatment of blood pressure and hypertension.

Further reading

Beevers DG. The 40th anniversary of the publication in 1964 of the first trial of the treatment of uncomplicated, severe hypertension by Hamilton, Thompson and Wisniewski. *J Hum Hypertens* 2004; **18**: 831–3.

Shevchenko YL, Tsitlik JE. 90th anniversary of the development by Nikolai S Korotkoff of the auscultatory method of measuring blood pressure. *Circulation* 1996; **94**: 116–18.

2. Blood pressure and hypertension

Blood pressure and cardiovascular risk
Prevalence of hypertension
Aetiology of hypertension

Blood pressure and cardiovascular risk

Hypertension is a common problem and a major preventable cardiovascular risk factor. Worldwide prevalence estimates for hypertension may be as high as a billion individuals, with deaths attributable to hypertension estimated to be approximately 1.7 million deaths per year. The prevalence (and incidence) of hypertension and associated morbidity and mortality are likely to rise with the increasing epidemic of obesity and as the population ages.

In the vast majority, hypertension is asymptomatic until complications occur. These complications include cerebrovascular disease, heart disease, peripheral vascular disease, renal failure and retinopathy – target organ damage. The benefit of blood pressure (BP) lowering is now well established, but the 'rule of halves' still dominates – roughly half of patients with hypertension are identified; only half of them are actually treated; and only half of these have adequate blood pressure control (Figure 2.1).

> Complications of hypertension include stroke, heart disease, peripheral vascular disease, renal failure and retinopathy

Defining hypertension and cardiovascular risk

Hypertension can be defined pragmatically as 'that level of BP above which the use of antihypertensive treatment does more good than harm'. This level will vary from patient to patient and balances the risks of untreated hypertension with those of long-term exposure to antihypertensive drugs and their side-effects. Hence, the diagnosis and treatment of hypertension must be individualized – the higher the patient's cardiovascular disease (CVD) risk, the greater the (absolute) benefit of BP reduction and the lower the threshold for BP treatment will be accordingly.

Indeed, this recognition of high BP in the context of a patient's overall CVD risk is central to the current recommendations by the second Joint British Societies guidelines, which advise antihypertensive treatment based on the 10-year CVD risk (replacing the previous coronary heart disease (CHD) risk) of ≥ 20% according to the current Joint British Societies risk assessment chart (Figure 2.2, inside front cover). There is a strong 'additive' effect of other risk factors such as diabetes, hyperlipidaemia, smoking and gender to the overall risk profile and thus a multifactorial approach should be considered. The charts are based on the Framingham risk function and specify three levels of 10-year CVD risk: ≥30%, ≥20% and ≤10%, which are equivalent to a CHD

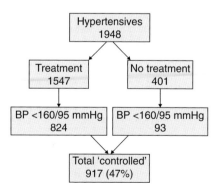

Figure 2.1
Hypertension in general practice in England, illustrating the 'rule of halves'. (Adapted from Poulter *et al*. *Blood Pressure* 1996; **5**: 209–15.)

risk of 23%, 15% and 8% respectively. These three groups are represented by three colour bands on the chart for easy use. The information needed to assess scores is shown in Table 2.1.

<table>
<tr><td colspan="2">Table 2.1
Use of the Joint British Societies CVD risk chart (see inside front cover)</td></tr>
<tr><td>Information needed:</td><td>Age
Sex
Systolic BP (mmHg)
Smoking status
Serum cholesterol (any units)
HDL cholesterol (same units as serum cholesterol)</td></tr>
</table>

The 10-year absolute CVD risk now replaces the CHD risk assessment. The CVD end-points include fatal/non-fatal myocardial infarction or angina plus stroke (fatal/non-fatal stroke and intracerebral haemorrhage) or transient ischaemic attack. Diabetes status is no longer included into the risk chart as most patients with diabetes have estimated 10-year CVD risk of ≥20%, and therefore considered at high risk.

Blood pressure should be considered in the context of overall cardiovascular risk

From a population perspective, hypertension is defined as sustained systolic BP between 140 and 159 mmHg or sustained diastolic BP between 90 and 99 mmHg. The British Hypertension Society (BHS) and the American Joint National Committee on prevention, detection, evaluation, and treatment of high BP (JNC-VII) guidelines are concordant in this regard. However, the broader blood pressure classification remains divergent between guidelines (see Table 2.3).

Hypertension and cardiovascular risk

There almost appears to be a dose–response relationship between hypertension and the risk of stroke or CHD; conversely, the reduction of BP by antihypertensive treatment reduces the risk of stroke and heart attacks (Figure 2.3).

In 1990, MacMahon et al. analysed nine prospective longitudinal observational studies from North America and Europe consisting of untreated middle-aged and predominantly (96%) male populations, totalling 4.2 million person-years of observation. After a mean follow-up of 10 years, this meta-analysis confirmed the positive, continuous, independent association of stroke and coronary risk with high BP throughout its range. The data suggest that a 5–6 mmHg reduction in the average level of diastolic BP would be associated with an approximately 40% reduction in stroke and a 20–25% reduction in CHD. Crucially, there was no evidence of a threshold between 'normal' BP and the pressure associated with higher risk. Furthermore, there was very little evidence in untreated populations of a so-called 'J-curve', where increased risk might be seen in individuals with low BPs. A more recent meta-analysis of 61 prospective studies by Lewington et al. reaffirms this dose–response relationship between blood pressure and cardiovascular mortality.

Reducing the average level of diastolic BP by 5–6 mmHg would give a 40% reduction in stroke and a 20–25% reduction in CHD

A lower level of risk appears to be present in women, at least below the age of 55 years. Also, in the Eastern Stroke and Coronary Heart Disease Collaborative Research Group study (1998) a different ratio between heart attacks and strokes is seen among Far Eastern populations.

In the Multiple Risk Factor Intervention Trial, a cross-tabulation of systolic and diastolic BPs found that relative risk of CHD would increase progressively as follows:

- 1.0 with optimal levels of BP (regular systolic BP <120 mmHg, diastolic BP <80 mmHg)
- 3.23 in isolated diastolic hypertension (diastolic BP >100 mmHg, systolic BP <120 mmHg)

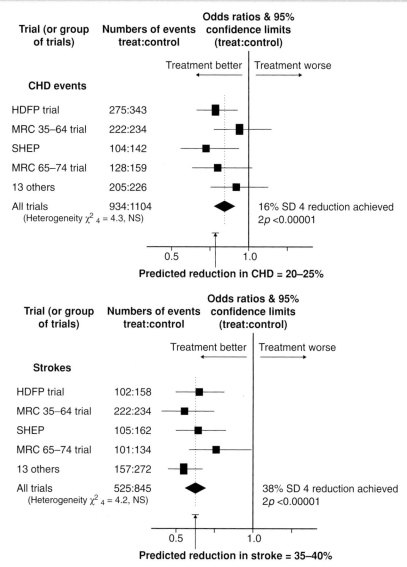

Figure 2.3
The effect of treating hypertension on the risk of suffering from coronary heart disease or stroke. CHD, coronary heart disease.

- 4.19 in people with isolated systolic hypertension (systolic BP >160 mmHg and diastolic BP <80 mmHg)
- 4.57 in those with a combined increase of both systolic and diastolic BP (systolic BP >160 mmHg, diastolic BP >100 mmHg).

This is illustrated in Figure 2.4. The corresponding rise of stroke risk is also shown.

There has been some debate on the relative importance of systolic and diastolic blood pressure, but in practice systolic blood pressure

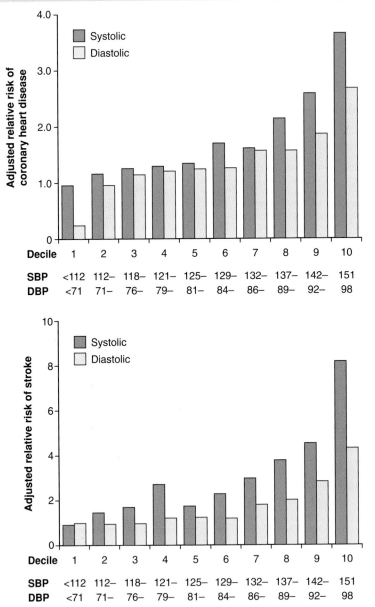

Figure 2.4
How increasing systolic and diastolic blood pressures affect the relative risk of coronary heart disease and stroke. SBP, systolic blood pressure; DBP, diastolic blood pressure. (Adapted from Stamler *et al. Arch Int Med* 1993; **153**: 598–615; He *et al. J Hypertens* 1999; **17**: 7–13.)

should be regarded as the more important. In epidemiological studies both systolic and diastolic blood pressure are important risk factors for cardiovascular disease. Certainly,

systolic blood pressure is a better predictor of cardiovascular mortality and morbidity even correcting for underlying diastolic blood pressure. Figure 2.4 clearly shows the greater effect of systolic blood pressure compared to diastolic on relative risk of CHD.

Geoffrey Rose and the population approach to cardiovascular risk

In a population, BP is a continuous variable, distributed in a roughly normal (or Gaussian) manner. There are not two separate groups of individuals (that is, those with and without hypertension) but a continuous range of BP from the lowest to the highest, with the majority of individuals falling somewhere in the middle. Although those with very high blood pressures are individually at very high risk of stroke and CHD, there are relatively few of them. Treating all these patients with severe hypertension would have little impact on the number of strokes and heart attacks occurring in the population as a whole, as most strokes and heart attacks occur in those with only mildly elevated or even normal BP. On the other hand, small reductions in BP of the population as a whole may result in greater numbers of cardiovascular events in the population. This population strategy is based on the axiom by the British epidemiologist Geoffrey Rose that 'a large number of people at small risk may give rise to more cases than a small number of people at high risk'.

> BP is a continuous variable distributed in a fairly normal manner. There are not two groups – people with and without hypertension – but a continuous range of BPs with most people falling somewhere in the middle

The 'population approach' to managing hypertension suggests that reducing the mean BP of the population as a whole by only a few mmHg using public health measures (such as reducing salt intake and increasing exercise) would significantly reduce the rate of stroke and CHD when compared to a strategy of achieving large reductions in BP in only a few individuals with severe hypertension.

However, contemporary medical practice has evolved from a single risk factor approach to an emphasis on CVD risk, which incorporates the assessment of multiple risk factors. This led to a recent re-examination of Rose's classic axiom by Manuel and colleagues. They reported on the estimated effectiveness of the population strategy compared to a single risk factor approach (in this case, targeting lipid-lowering treatment in patients with high cholesterol levels) and a cardiovascular risk approach (targeting treatment at patients with the highest CVD risk). Based on their results, the strategy of targeting individuals at highest CVD risk was by far the most effective. Their study lends support to the current recommendations for a CVD risk guided approach to the management of patients with cardiovascular risk factors, including hypertension.

> The strategy of targeting individuals at highest CVD risk is by far the most effective

Prevalence of hypertension

Using a definition of a systolic BP >140 mmHg or a diastolic BP >90 mmHg or current treatment with antihypertensive medication, the prevalence of hypertension in the US population varies from 4% in 18–29-year-olds to 65% in those aged 80 years and over. Data from the Birmingham Factory Screen project are illustrated in Figure 2.5. This shows the rise in blood pressure with age, as well as ethnic differences.

Nevertheless, hypertension is not distributed evenly in the community, and even in the UK there are variations with geography. For example, in a survey of 24 large towns, the lowest mean BP was found in Shrewsbury, while the highest was in Dunfermline where the BP (systolic/diastolic) was on average 17/11 mmHg higher.

Systolic blood pressure also rises steadily with increasing age, and the prevalence of hypertension including isolated systolic hypertension (systolic BP $\geq$ 160/diastolic BP <90 mmHg) is more than 50% in those aged

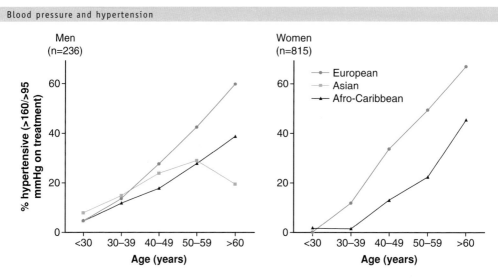

Men
(n=236)

Women
(n=815)

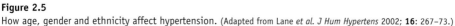

Figure 2.5
How age, gender and ethnicity affect hypertension. (Adapted from Lane *et al. J Hum Hypertens* 2002; **16**: 267–73.)

over 60 years. Isolated systolic hypertension is the predominant form of hypertension found in the older population (Figure 2.6). In premenopausal women, hypertension has a lower prevalence in women than in men, but beyond the age of 65 years, the mean systolic BP in women at least approaches that seen in older men, and has occasionally been reported

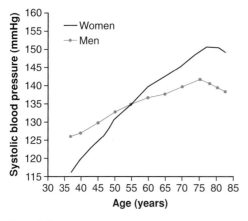

Figure 2.6
Cross-sectional age trend of systolic hypertension in men and women. (Adapted from Kannel WB. *Am Heart J* 1999; **138**: s 205.)

to be even higher, with overall prevalence estimated at 30–50% in women aged 65 years or older. Indeed, hypertension is an important contributor to morbidity and mortality in postmenopausal women in Western countries (Figure 2.7).

Many patients with 'high normal' blood pressure levels will progress to overt hypertension. In the Framingham Heart Study, 9845 non-hypertensive patients were followed up for 4 years, and their blood pressures were initially classified as: optimum (SBP<120 and DBP<80 mmHg), normal (SBP 120–9 or DBP 80–4 mmHg) or high normal (SBP 130–9 or DBP 85–9 mmHg). The proportions progressing to >140/90 are illustrated in Table 2.2.

These findings support recommendations for monitoring individuals with high normal BP once a year, and monitoring those with normal blood pressure every 2 years, and they emphasize the importance of weight control as a measure for primary prevention of hypertension. Indeed, the American guidelines highlight this increased risk of developing hypertension among individuals with blood pressure of 120–139 mmHg systolic and 80–89

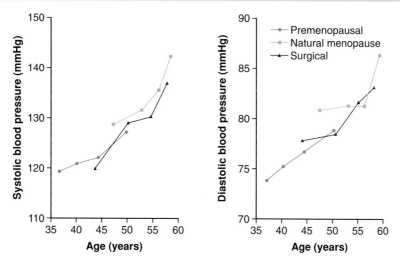

Figure 2.7
The influence of the menopause on blood pressure. The adjusted blood pressure rise with age was steeper in postmenopausal women. (Adapted from Staesson *et al. J Hum Hypertens* 1989; **3**: 427–33.)

mmHg diastolic with the designation of 'pre-hypertension' (Table 2.3).

Aetiology of hypertension

The vast majority (>95%) of patients with hypertension have primary or essential (idiopathic) hypertension, where there is no immediate underlying cause (Figure 2.8). This definition is somewhat misleading in that all hypertension clearly has a cause, albeit one due to the interplay of complex genetic and environmental factors.

Table 2.2
Progression to hypertension in the Framingham Heart Study (Adapted from Vasan *et al. Lancet* 2001; **358**: 1682–6)

	Baseline BP (mmHg)	% progressing to >140/90 mmHg over 4 years
Age 35–64	<120 and <80	5.1%
	120–9 or 80–4	18.1%
	130–9 or 85–9	39.4%
Age 65–94	<120 and <80	18.5%
	120–9 or 80–4	29.2%
	130–9 or 85–9	52.5%

Even in so-called 'essential hypertension', lifestyle influences such as salt and potassium intake, alcohol, dietary factors and exercise can contribute to raised BP, as do gender, ethnic origin and body mass index. Acute stress can cause a rise in BP, but there is little evidence of

Table 2.3 (a)
The definitions and classification of BP levels (BHS-IV, 2004)

Category	Systolic BP (mmHg)	Diastolic BP (mmHg)
Optimal	<120	<80
Normal	<130	<85
High normal	130–139	85–89
Grade 1 hypertension (mild)	140–159	90–99
Grade 2 hypertension (moderate)	160–179	100–109
Grade 3 hypertension (severe)	≥180	≥110
Isolated systolic hypertension:		
Grade 1	140–159	<90
Grade 2	≥160	<90

When a patient's systolic blood pressure and diastolic blood pressure fall into different categories, the higher category should apply. BP, blood pressure.

Table 2.3 (b)
Classification of blood pressure in adults (JNC-VII)

Blood pressure classification	Systolic blood pressure (mmHg)	Diastolic blood pressure (mmHg)
Normal	<120	And <80
Pre-hypertension	120–139	Or 80–89
Stage 1 hypertension	140–159	Or 90–99
Stage 2 hypertension	≥160	Or ≥100

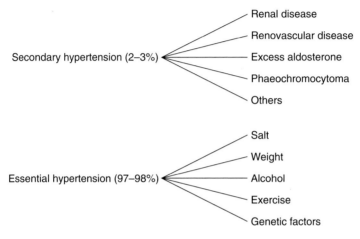

Figure 2.8
Essential and secondary hypertension.

a causal effect of chronic stress on BP. The so-called 'Barker hypothesis' suggests that fetal influences, particularly birth weight, may be a determinant of adult BP. For example, small babies are more likely to have high BP as adolescents and to be hypertensive as adults.

The majority of patients with hypertension have primary or essential hypertension

In a small minority of patients, hypertension is 'secondary', or due to an underlying disease usually involving the kidneys or endocrine system (see Chapter 4). Effective treatment of the underlying condition can sometimes abolish the hypertension.

Further reading

Colhoun HM, Dong W, Poulter NR. Blood pressure screening, management and control in England: results from the health survey for England 1994. *J Hypertens* 1998; **16**: 747–52.

Eastern Stroke and Coronary Heart Disease Collaborative Research Group. Blood pressure, cholesterol, and stroke in eastern Asia. *Lancet* 1998; **352**: 1801–7.

JBS 2: Joint British Societies' guidelines on prevention of cardiovascular disease in clinical practice. *Heart* 2005; **91**: 1–52.

Lewington S, Clarke R, Qizilbash N, *et al.* Age-specific relevance of usual blood pressure to vascular mortality: a meta-analysis of individual data for one million adults in 61 prospective studies. Prospective Studies Collaboration. *Lancet* 2002; **360**: 1903–13.

Manuel DG, Lim J, Tanuseputro P, *et al.* Revisiting Rose: strategies for reducing coronary heart disease. *BMJ* 2006; **332**: 659–62.

Rosenthal T, Oparil S. Hypertension in women. *J Hum Hypertens* 2000; **14**: 691–704.

Seedat YK. Hypertension in developing nations in sub-Saharan Africa. *J Hum Hypertens* 2000; **14**: 739–47.

Seventh Report of the Joint National Committee on Prevention, Detection, Evaluation and Treatment of High Blood Pressure. *Hypertension* 2003; **42**: 1206–52.

Singh RB, Suh IL, Singh VP, *et al*. Hypertension and stroke in Asia: prevalence, control and strategies in developing countries for prevention. *J Hum Hypertens* 2000; **14**: 749–63.

Ueshima H, Zhang XH, Choudhury SR. Epidemiology of hypertension in China and Japan. *J Hum Hypertens* 2000; **14**: 765–9.

Williams B, Poulter NR, Brown MJ, *et al*. Guidelines for management of hypertension: report of the fourth working party of the British Hypertension Society. *J Hum Hypertens* 2004; **18**: 139–85.

World Health Organisation. International Society Guidelines for the Management of Hypertension. Guidelines Subcommittee. *J Hypertens* 1999; **17**: 151–83.

3. Pathophysiology

Cardiac output and peripheral resistance
Arterial stiffness
Renin–angiotensin system
Autonomic nervous system
Hypercoagulability
Endothelial dysfunction
Other factors

The pathophysiology of hypertension is complex, and the subject of much uncertainty. In most cases (95%), no single identifiable cause is found and the condition is labelled 'essential hypertension'. A small number of patients (between 2% and 5%) have an underlying secondary disease as the cause of their hypertension.

Many physiological mechanisms are involved in the maintenance of normal blood pressure (BP), and pathophysiological abnormalities in these systems might play a part in the development of essential hypertension. The factors that influence BP include:

- salt intake
- physical activity
- obesity and insulin resistance
- the renin–angiotensin system
- the sympathetic nervous system.

Additional factors proposed include:

- genetics
- endothelial dysfunction (including changes in mediators, such as endothelin and nitric oxide)
- hypercoagulability

- low birth weight
- intrauterine nutrition
- neurovascular anomalies.

Their relative roles may differ between individuals and ethnic groups. For example, there is a high prevalence of insulin resistance in the peoples of South Asia, which can be associated with obesity, diabetes and lipid abnormalities – the so-called 'metabolic syndrome'.

> Hypertension has a complex pathophysiology with most cases exhibiting no clear single identifiable cause, though abnormalities in the physiological mechanisms involved in maintaining normal BP may play a part in its development

Cardiac output and peripheral resistance

Normal BP depends upon a balance between the cardiac output and peripheral vascular resistance. In essential hypertension, cardiac output is normal but peripheral resistance is raised. The latter is determined by the state of small arterioles, the walls of which contain smooth muscle cells, and not by large arteries or the capillaries.

In early hypertension, especially in younger patients, BP elevation may be caused by a raised cardiac output related to sympathetic overactivity (peripheral resistance is not raised). Compensatory vasoconstriction of resistance vessels (arterioles) prevents the raised pressure being transmitted to the capillary bed where it would substantially affect cell homeostasis. This initial response of the vasculature to mild to moderate elevations of blood pressure is probably mediated by endogenous vasoconstrictors such as angiotensin and endothelin. However, prolonged smooth muscle constriction induces structural changes in these arterioles, with vessel wall thickening possibly mediated by angiotensin, which leads to an irreversible rise in peripheral resistance. The intracellular calcium concentration found in smooth muscle cells is responsible for this contraction, and explains the vasodilatory effect of calcium channel blockers.

> In very early hypertension, raised BP may be caused by a raised cardiac output related to sympathetic overactivity

Auto-regulation in hypertension

In chronic hypertension, the lower limit of auto-regulation of cerebral blood flow is shifted towards higher BPs, with impairment of the tolerance to acute hypotension. For example, in normotensive subjects, the upper limit of auto-regulation can be a mean arterial pressure of 120 mmHg (or about 160/100 mmHg), but in individuals whose vessels are hypertrophied by longstanding hypertension, it may be substantially higher.

In very severe hypertension, such as is seen in hypertensive emergencies, intense peripheral vasoconstriction results in a rapid rise in BP and a vicious cycle of events that includes ischaemia of the brain and peripheral organs. This ischaemia stimulates neurohormone and cytokine release, exacerbating the vasoconstriction and-ischaemia, further increasing BP and leading to target organ damage. In addition, myointimal proliferation in the vasculature can make the situation worse, as may disseminated intravascular coagulation. Furthermore, renal ischaemia leads to the activation of the renin–angiotensin system causing a further rise in BP and microvascular damage.

With rapid and severe rises in BP, the process of auto-regulation fails, leading to a rise in pressure in the arterioles and capillaries, causing vascular damage. This disruption of the endothelium allows plasma constituents (including fibrinoid material) to enter the vessel wall, narrowing or obliterating the lumen

in many tissue beds. The level at which fibrinoid necrosis occurs is dependent upon the baseline BP. In the cerebral circulation, this can lead to the development of cerebral oedema and the clinical picture of hypertensive encephalopathy.

In addition to protecting the tissues against the effects of hypertension, auto-regulation maintains perfusion during the treatment of hypertension via arterial and arteriolar vasodilatation.

However, excessive falls in BP below the auto-regulatory range can lead to organ ischaemia. The arteriolar hypertrophy induced by chronic hypertension means target organ ischaemia will occur at a higher BP than in previously normotensive subjects (Figure 3.1).

> Rapid and severe rises in BP can cause auto-regulation to fail, followed by vascular damage caused by a rise in pressure in the arterioles and capillaries

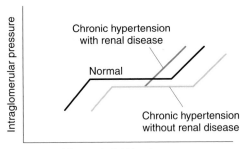

Figure 3.1
Auto-regulatory mechanism to maintain relatively constant organ blood flow across a range of blood pressures. Intraglomerular pressure (renal blood flow) is illustrated in this case, with a rightward shift in the auto-regulatory curve (light blue line). Hence, rapid and excessive blood pressure reduction into the 'normal' range may compromise renal function. Also highlighted here is the narrowed auto-regulation range (dark blue line) in patients with renal disease (more sensitive to increased blood pressure). (Adapted from Palmer BF. Renal dysfunction complicating the treatment of hypertension. *N Engl J Med* 2002; **347**: 1256–61.)

Arterial stiffness

Arterial stiffness describes the mechanical properties of the arterial system. These mechanical properties can be inferred by various methods, including quantification of compliance (or distensibility) and pulse wave velocity (the time taken for a pressure wave to travel a known distance). The latter is widely used to characterize the 'stiffness' of the artery, based on the principle that the pulse wave travels faster in stiffer arteries.

In older patients and patients with hypertension and diabetes, changes in the arterial wall (e.g. elastin to collagen ratio and glycation of connective tissue) result in 'stiffening' of the arterial tree. The consequent increase in pulse wave velocity is associated with earlier pulse wave reflection at branch points. The earlier return of these reflected waves augments the systolic instead of diastolic pressure wave, resulting in increased systolic pressure and reduced diastolic pressure in the central arterial circulation (aorta and large vessels).

The recent CAFÉ study (a substudy of the ASCOT) demonstrated significantly higher central arterial blood pressure in the atenolol-based group compared to the amlodipine-based antihypertensive regime, despite similar blood pressure reduction measured at the brachial artery. These differences may explain the higher rates of cardiovascular events with atenolol treatment in the ASCOT study.

Renin–angiotensin system

The renin–angiotensin system is probably the most important of the endocrine systems controlling BP. The kidney's juxtaglomerular apparatus secretes renin in response to glomerular underperfusion or a reduced salt intake. Renin is also released in response to stimulation from the sympathetic nervous system. Renin is responsible for converting renin substrate (angiotensinogen) to angiotensin I, a physiologically inactive substance that is rapidly converted to angiotensin II in the lungs by angiotensin-converting enzyme (ACE). Angiotensin II is a potent vasoconstrictor and thus causes a rise in BP. It also stimulates the release of aldosterone from the adrenal zona glomerulosa, which results in both sodium and water retention (Figure 3.2).

There are also important non-circulating 'local' renin–angiotensin epicrine or paracrine systems in the kidney, the heart and the arterial tree which also control BP and may have important roles in regulating regional blood flow.

Although the circulating renin–angiotensin system may have a pathophysiological role, this endocrine system is not a direct or the sole cause of hypertension. This is especially evident in the elderly or in Afro-Caribbean patients, who have low levels of renin and angiotensin II; drugs which block the renin–angiotensin system are less effective in such patient groups (Table 3.1). None the less, the renin–angiotensin system is an important target for the treatment of hypertension.

Table 3.1

Drugs which block the renin system (beta-blockers, ACE inhibitors and angiotensin receptor blockers) tend to be less effective in patients with low renin and angiotensin levels

Low renin states:	
Anephrics	Older patients
Patients with Conn's syndrome	Afro-Caribbean patients
Patients with liquorice-induced hypertension	Patients with type 2 diabetes

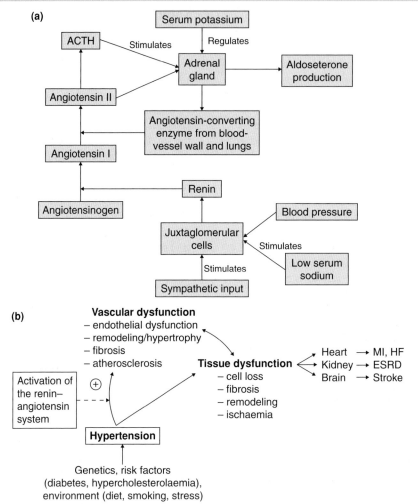

Figure 3.2
(a) The renin–angiotensin–aldosterone system. (b) The renin–angiotensin drives the pathology in hypertension. ACTH, adrenocorticotropic hormone; ESRD, end stage renal disease; HF, heart failure; MI, myocardial infarction. (Adapted from Weir *et al*. *Am J Hypertens* 1999; **12**: 205S–35; Timmermans *et al*. *Pharmacol Rev* 1993; **45**: 205–51.)

Autonomic nervous system

The autonomic nervous system plays an important role in the pathophysiology of hypertension, and is key to maintaining a normal BP. For example, sympathetic nervous system stimulation can cause both arteriolar constriction and arteriolar dilation, depending on whether or not the receptors are excitatory or inhibitory.

The autonomic nervous system is important in the mediation of short-term changes in BP in response to stress and physical exercise. However, adrenaline (epinephrine) and noradrenaline (norepinephrine) may not have a clear role in the aetiology of hypertension, though drugs used for the treatment of hypertension do block the sympathetic nervous system and have a well-established therapeutic role. There is more likely to be a complex interaction between the autonomic nervous system and the various neuroendocrine systems (including the renin–angiotensin system), together with other factors, including circulating sodium volume.

> The autonomic nervous system has a central role in hypertension pathophysiology, maintaining a normal BP and mediating short-term changes in BP in response to stress and physical exercise

Hypercoagulability

While the blood vessels are exposed to high pressures in hypertension, paradoxically, the main complications of hypertension (stroke and myocardial infarction) are thrombotic rather than haemorrhagic – the so-called thrombotic paradox of hypertension (or 'Birmingham paradox') (Figure 3.3). Increasing evidence suggests that patients with hypertension demonstrate abnormalities of:

- vessel walls (endothelial dysfunction or damage)
- blood constituents (abnormal levels of haemostatic factors, platelet activation and fibrinolysis)
- blood flow (rheology, viscosity and flow reserve).

The fulfilment of the three components of Virchow's triad for thrombogenesis suggests that hypertension confers a prothrombotic or

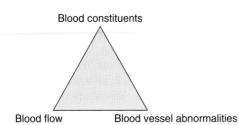

Blood constituents

Blood flow   Blood vessel abnormalities

Figure 3.3
Virchow's triad of thrombogenesis. Abnormalities of all three components of Virchow's triad are present in hypertension; hypertension confers a prothrombotic state.

hypercoagulable state, which appears to be related to the degree or severity of target organ damage. These abnormalities can be related to long-term prognosis and in addition, may be altered by antihypertensive treatment.

Endothelial dysfunction

Vascular endothelial cells play a key role in cardiovascular regulation by producing a number of potent local vasoactive agents, including the vasodilator molecule nitric oxide (NO) and the vasoconstrictor peptide endothelin. Dysfunction of the endothelium, therefore, may lead to alteration in vascular tone and arterial blood pressure. Indeed, endothelial damage or dysfunction is well-described in human essential hypertension.

Modulation of the endothelial function is an attractive therapeutic option in attempting to minimize some of the important complications of hypertension. Clinically effective antihypertensive therapy appears to restore impaired production of nitric oxide, but does not seem to restore the impaired endothelium-dependent vascular relaxation or vascular response to endothelial receptors. This indicates that such endothelial dysfunction is primary and becomes irreversible once the hypertensive process has become established.

Vasoactive substances

Many vasoactive systems and mechanisms that affect sodium transport and vascular tone are involved in maintaining normal BP. For example, endothelin is a powerful, vascular, endothelial vasoconstrictor, which may produce a 'salt-sensitive' rise in BP. It also activates local renin–angiotensin systems. Bradykinin is a potent vasodilator, which is inactivated by an angiotensin-converting enzyme. Consequently, treatment with ACE inhibitors may exert some of their effect by blocking bradykinin inactivation.

Endothelial-derived relaxant factor, which is now known to be nitric oxide (NO), is produced by arterial and venous endothelium and diffuses through the vessel wall into the smooth muscle causing vasodilatation. The production of NO also modulates the thrombotic balance and may limit the prothrombotic tendencies in hypertension described above.

Nevibolol, a novel beta-blocker with NO-modulating effects, has been shown to be an effective blood pressure-lowering agent, but it is unclear if the NO-modulating effects confer any additional benefits. It is possible that this property may limit the side-effects associated with beta-blockers, for example impotence, which is common with other beta-blockers.

Atrial natriuretic peptide (ANP) is a hormone secreted from the atria of the heart in response to increased blood volume. The effect of ANP is to increase sodium and water excretion from the kidney. Modulation of this hormone has been a target for agents such as omapatrilat, a vasopeptidase inhibitor, with the aim of treating hypertension and heart failure. However, data from randomized studies were disappointing, emphasizing the complexity and unpredictability of neurohormonal modulation.

> Many vasoactive systems and sodium transport-affecting mechanisms are involved in maintaining normal BP, such as endothelin and bradykinin

Other factors
Angiogenesis

Abnormal angiogenesis has been demonstrated in hypertensive animal models as well as in different stages of hypertension in humans. In hypertension, there seems to be an impaired ability for vascular growth resulting from structural alteration of the microvascular network, which includes capillary rarefaction, increased arteriolar length and tortuosity. These alterations in the microvasculature appear at very early stages of hypertension, and increasing evidence points to the possibility

that abnormal angiogenesis may contribute causally to hypertension.

Sodium transport

The transport of sodium across vascular smooth muscle cell walls could influence BP via its interrelationship with calcium transport.

Insulin sensitivity

Several 'classic' risk factors, such as obesity, glucose intolerance, diabetes mellitus and hyperlipidaemia, tend to cluster together. The frequent association of these risk factors led to the suggestion of a clinical syndrome, now termed the metabolic syndrome. Obesity and insulin resistance (generally defined by high levels of insulin in the face of normal or high glucose levels), is widely regarded as a central feature of this syndrome. However, some hypertensive patients who are not obese display resistance to insulin. The metabolic syndrome, which is especially prevalent in South Asians (who are at high risk of ischaemic heart disease), could explain why the hazards of cardiovascular risk are synergistic or multiplicative rather than simply additive. In view of the well-documented associations between these risk factors, the presence of hypertension should prompt the search for other risk factors (e.g. diabetes and dyslipidaemia).

Genetic factors

Human essential hypertension is a complex, multifactorial, quantitative trait under polygenic control. Over the last decade several strategies have been used to dissect the genetic determinants of hypertension. Separate genes and genetic factors have been linked to the development of essential hypertension, but multiple genes probably contribute to the development of the disorder in a particular individual. It is rare that a specific genetic mutation can cause hypertension and the condition is twice as common in subjects with one or two hypertensive parents. Genetic factors account for approximately 30% of the variation in BP in various populations.

In the quest for a gene (or genes) for hypertension, the study of rare monogenic forms of hypertension has been the most successful. Attempts to identify the multiple genes involved in the more common polygenic form of hypertension have been much more difficult. Many laboratories use rat models of genetic hypertension where some of the complexity of studying human hypertension can be removed, but whether such information can be applied to large populations of hypertensive patients remains debatable. Numerous crosses between hypertensive and normotensive rat strains have produced several quantitative trait loci for blood pressure and other related phenotypes such as left ventricular hypertrophy, stroke, insulin resistance and kidney failure.

Intrauterine influences

Fetal influences, particularly birth weight, may be a determinant of BP in adult life, although the precise pathophysiological mechanisms are still uncertain. For example, babies with a low birth weight are more likely to have higher BPs during adolescence and to be hypertensive as adults.

The Barker hypothesis states that small-for-age babies are also more likely to have metabolic abnormalities that have been associated with the later development of hypertension and cardiovascular disease, such as insulin resistance, diabetes mellitus, hyperlipidaemia and abdominal obesity. This hypothesis has been applied to the South Asian population to explain the increased cardiovascular risk in this population.

Another interpretation suggests that genetic factors may explain the Barker hypothesis. For example, mothers with above average BP in pregnancy give birth to smaller babies who subsequently develop above average BP themselves and eventually hypertension. It is entirely likely that the similarity of BPs in mother and child are genetic and in a modern 'healthy' society, unrelated to intrauterine under-nutrition.

Further reading

Blann AD, Lip GYH. The endothelium in atherothrombotic disease: assessment of function, mechanisms and clinical implications. *Blood Coag Fibrinolys* 1998; **9**: 297–306.

Eriksson JG, Forsen T, Tuomilehto J, *et al.* Early growth and coronary heart disease in later life: longitudinal study. *BMJ* 2001; **322**: 949–53.

Gibbons GH. The pathophysiology of hypertension: the importance of angiotensin II in cardiovascular remodeling. *Am J Hypertens* 1998; **11**: 177S–181S.

Lee WK, Padmanabhan S, Dominiczak AF. Genetics of hypertension: from experimental models to clinical applications. *J Hum Hypertens* 2000; **14**: 631–47.

Le Noble FAC, Stassen FRM, Hacking WJG, *et al.* Angiogenesis and hypertension. *J Hypertens* 1998; **16**: 1563–72.

Lip GYH. Hypertension and the prothrombotic state. *J Hum Hypertens* 2000; **14**: 687–90.

Lip GYH, Blann AD. Does hypertension confer a prothrombotic state? Virchow's triad revisited. *Circulation* 2000; **101**: 218–20.

Nicholls MG, Robertson JI. The renin–angiotensin system in the year 2000. *J Hum Hypertens* 2000; **14**: 649–66.

Roseboom TJ, van der Meulen JH, van Montfrans GA, *et al.* Maternal nutrition during gestation and blood pressure in later life. *J Hypertens* 2001; **19**: 29–34.

Ross R. The pathogenesis of atherosclerosis: a perspective for the 1990s. *Nature* 1993; **362**: 801–9.

Safar ME, Levy BI, Struijker-Boudier H. Current perspectives on arterial stiffness and pulse pressure in hypertension and cardiovascular disease. *Circulation* 2003; **107**: 2864–9.

Sagnella GA. Atrial natriuretic peptide mimetics and vasopeptidase inhibitors. *Cardiovasc Res* 2001; **51**: 416–28.

Schlaich MP, Schmieder RE. Left ventricular hypertrophy and its regression: pathophysiology and therapeutic approach: focus on treatment by antihypertensive agents. *Am J Hypertens* 1998; **11**: 1394–404.

Spieker LE, Noll G, Ruschitzka FT, *et al.* Working under pressure: the vascular endothelium in arterial hypertension. *J Hum Hypertens* 2000; **14**: 617–30.

4. Target organ damage

Cerebrovascular disease
Heart
Large vessel arterial disease
Kidney and renal failure
Retinopathy

Table 4.1
Definite and possible risk factors for stroke

Definite	Possible
Hypertension	Lipid level
Atrial fibrillation	Salt consumption
Coronary heart disease	Low potassium diet
Diabetes	Low vitamin C diet
TIA	Fibrinogen
Smoking	
Carotid disease	
Alcohol excess	

The natural history of high blood pressure (BP) can be regarded as having two stages. Initially, hypertension can develop as a risk factor, without significant local organ damage or symptoms. Later, this can shift towards significant target organ damage with cardiovascular symptoms. This can manifest itself as blocking effects (atherothrombotic plaques causing coronary, cerebrovascular or peripheral artery disease) or 'bursting' effects (cerebral haemorrhage, aortic dissection or heart failure).

Cerebrovascular disease

Stroke is one of the most devastating consequences of hypertension, and can result in significant disability as well as in premature death. Definite and possible stroke risk factors are summarized in Table 4.1.

Strokes account for about 12% of all deaths, and about 25% of all strokes occur in patients younger than 65 years. After standardizing for age, men aged 40–59 years with a systolic BP of 160–180 mmHg are approximately four times more likely to suffer a stroke during the next eight years when compared to men with a systolic BP of 140–159 mmHg. An average reduction of just 9/5 mmHg in BP results in a 34% reduction in the incidence of stroke

whereas a reduction of 19/10 mmHg results in a 56% lower incidence of stroke.

Strokes account for 12% of deaths, with 25% of all strokes affecting the under-65 age group. Men with a systolic BP of 160–180 mmHg are around four times more likely to have a stroke than men with a systolic BP of 140–159 mmHg

In patients with hypertension, about 80% of strokes are ischaemic, caused by intra-arterial thrombosis or embolization from the heart and large arteries. The remaining 20% are due to haemorrhagic causes, which may also be related to very high BP. In the UK 40% of all strokes are estimated to be linked to a systolic BP of 140 mmHg or more. The relation between prior blood pressure control and odds ratio for stroke is illustrated in Figure 4.1. Stroke recurrence after transient ischaemic attack (TIA) or minor stroke is also greater with higher blood pressures (Figure 4.2).

Strokes and the elderly

Elderly hypertensive patients are particularly prone to developing all types of stroke and often sustain multiple small, asymptomatic cerebral infarcts, leading to progressive loss of intellectual function and dementia. Indeed, the recent SYT-EUR study convincingly showed that treatment of isolated systolic hypertension, which is generally more frequent in the elderly, resulted in the prevention of dementia at follow-up (Table 4.2).

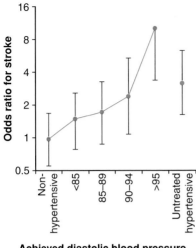

Figure 4.1
Prior blood pressure control and odds ratio for stroke.
(Adapted from Du *et al. Br Med J* 1997; **314**: 272–6.)

Table 4.2
The Syst-Eur dementia substudy (Adapted from Forette *et al. Lancet* 1998; **352**: 1347–51)

	Placebo	Active	p value
Number in trial	1180	1238	
All dementia	21	11	<0.05
Alzheimer's	15	8	NS
Mixed	4	3	NS
Vascular	2	0	NS

atrial fibrillation are additional to the risk of stroke. In the low risk arm of the third Stroke Prevention in Atrial Fibrillation study (SPAF-3), even a history of previous hypertension increased the risk of stroke nearly four-fold, despite aspirin therapy. In view of the significant risk of stroke, patients with hypertension and atrial fibrillation should be considered for anticoagulation.

Strokes and atrial fibrillation

Hypertension is also associated with an increased risk of atrial fibrillation, which is the most common sustained cardiac rhythm disorder. The presence of both hypertension and

Heart
Coronary heart disease

Fatal coronary heart disease (CHD) is seven times more common among hypertensives than a fatal stroke, and is the major population

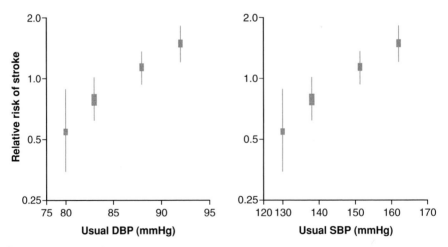

Figure 4.2
Stroke recurrence after transient ischaemic attack (TIA) or minor stroke. DBP, diastolic blood pressure; SBP, systolic blood pressure. (Adapted from Rogers *et al. Br Med J* 1996; **313**: 147.)

consequence of hypertension. Early trials of hypertension treatment provided convincing evidence for reductions in the risk of stroke but little evidence of benefit on coronary heart disease. However, these studies were not adequately powered to evaluate the impact of blood pressure treatment on CHD events. Indeed, subsequent larger controlled trials confirmed the benefit of blood pressure reduction on CHD events, although the reduction of coronary thrombosis is less impressive. Nevertheless, analysis of the large treatment trials suggests that adequate treatment of hypertension reduces the risk of heart attack by approximately 25%, although this is based on BP reduction with thiazides and beta-blockers, rather than the newer antihypertensive drugs.

Left ventricular hypertrophy

As a result of the increased afterload placed on the heart by high BP, the mass of the left ventricular muscle increases. While this is initially a compensatory response, increased muscle mass outstrips its oxygen supply. When left ventricular hypertrophy (LVH) is coupled with the reduced coronary vascular reserve in hypertension, it can result in myocardial ischaemia even with patent epicardial coronary arteries.

Thus, beyond a certain point, LVH secondary to hypertension becomes a major risk factor for myocardial infarction, stroke, congestive cardiac failure and sudden death. This increased risk is in addition to that imposed by hypertension itself. Hypertensives with LVH are also at an increased risk of developing cardiac arrhythmias (atrial fibrillation, ventricular arrhythmias) and atherosclerotic vascular disease (coronary and peripheral artery disease). Indeed, for a given level of BP, and if LVH is present, the prognosis is three or four times worse, especially for cardiac failure and stroke (Table 4.3).

Pathogenesis of LVH

The mechanisms promoting the development of LVH remain uncertain. The basic underlying mechanism may be an increase in ventricular wall stress and pressure workload on the left ventricle. Thus, with an increase in afterload as a result of hypertension, the heart responds with an increase in wall thickness. There is, however, a poor correlation between left ventricular wall thickness and BP. In addition, the pathogenesis of LVH has been shown to be influenced by demographic factors, such as age, sex, race and body habitus; exogenous factors, such as dietary salt intake and alcohol consumption; and neurohumoral substances, such as activity of the renin–angiotensin–aldosterone system, the sympathetic system, growth hormone and insulin. Several mechanisms have also been postulated for the role of the renin–angiotensin system in the pathogenesis of LVH. First,

Table 4.3
Relative risks of cardiovascular events and risk with increments in LV mass from Framingham data (Levy et al. Prognostic implications of echocardiographically determined left ventricular mass in the Framingham Heart Study. N Engl J Med 1990; **322**: 1561–6)

| | Relative risk (95%CI) for 50 g increase in LV mass | |
	Men	Women
CVD events	1.49(1.20–1.88)	1.57(1.20–2.04)
Cardiovascular mortality	1.73(1.19–2.52)	2.12(1.28–3.49)
Total mortality	1.49(1.14–1.94)	2.01(1.33–2.81)

All values have been adjusted for age, antihypertensive medications and standard CVD risk factors including blood pressure. LV, left ventricular; CVD, cardiovascular disease.

angiotensin II has direct and widespread vasoconstrictor actions, with effects on left ventricular afterload and myocardial ischaemia. Second, angiotensin II can also indirectly stimulate myocyte hypertrophy via its interaction with sympathetic tone, and in addition could be trophic to myocytes. This may stimulate fibroblastic proliferation and collagen formation; these factors are involved in the development of LVH (Table 4.4).

> The factors affecting the development of LVH remain unclear. The basic underlying mechanism may be an increase in ventricular wall stress and pressure workload on the left ventricle

Table 4.4
Possible adverse features of left ventricular hypertrophy

- Mismatch of blood supply and non-vascular tissue resulting in a relatively 'starved' subendocardial region
- Increased basal myocardial oxygen demand due to increased mass and wall stress
- A heightened likelihood of ventricular arrhythmias, perhaps related to the presence of fibrous tissue
- A markedly reduced coronary flow reserve, with abnormalities in the ability to dilate coronary arteries, resulting in increased cardiac ischaemia

Screening for LVH

A commonly used screening test for LVH in hypertensive patients is the 12-lead electrocardiogram (ECG). The usual criteria are those proposed by Sokolow and Lyon, that is, the sum of the S wave in lead V1 and the R wave in leads V5 or V6 on the ECG >35 mm. Nevertheless, LVH may be identified by electrocardiography in only 5–10% of hypertensive patients, while echocardiography is a far more sensitive investigation, identifying LVH in around 50% of untreated hypertensive patients. The various ECG criteria used for defining LVH are summarized in Table 4.5.

LVH and cardiac arrhythmias

LVH is also a risk factor for the development of cardiac arrhythmias, the most common being atrial fibrillation and ventricular arrhythmias. The presence of atrial fibrillation is important as this arrhythmia is associated with a five-fold increase in mortality and may often require long-term antiarrhythmic and antithrombotic therapy. Also, ventricular arrhythmias have important implications for the risk of sudden death in these patients. The mechanisms for sudden death are complex and may include malignant cardiac arrhythmias, including increased ventricular ectopics and nonsustained ventricular tachycardia. However, this risk of sudden death is independent of arterial pressure. Electrophysiological mechanisms for

Table 4.5
Electrocardiographic criteria for the diagnosis of left ventricular hypertrophy

Criterion	Measurement	Author(s) and year of description
R wave in aVL	R aVL	Sokolow and Lyon 1949
Sokolow–Lyon	SV1 + R (V5 or V6)	Sokolow and Lyon 1949
Cornell	RaVL + SV3	Casale et al. 1985
Cornell Voltage Duration Product	RaVL + SV3 × QRS duration	Molloy et al. 1992
Cornell/QRS II	RaVL + SV3/Total QRS voltage in lead II	Denarié et al. 1998
Lewis	RI − RIII + SIII − SI	Lewis 1914
RI + SIII	RI + SIII	Gubner and Ungerleider 1943

arrhythmogenesis in left ventricular hypertrophy (LVH) are summarized in Table 4.6.

Table 4.6
Electrophysiological mechanisms for arrhythmogenesis in left ventricular hypertrophy (LVH)

- Re-entry mechanisms related to myocardial fibrosis in LVH
- Myocardial ischaemic areas, perhaps related to reduced coronary reserve (as coronary artery disease is often not present)
- Ventricular myocyte stretching and arterial wall tension in the hypertrophied heart
- Increased sympathetic nervous system activity

LVH is a risk factor in developing cardiac arrhythmias, such as atrial fibrillation – associated with a five-fold increase in mortality – and ventricular arrhythmias

Heart failure as a complication of LVH

Heart failure is another complication commonly associated with LVH and hypertension. In the Framingham study, the presence of LVH on the ECG is associated with a substantially increased risk of heart failure. The way in which hypertension results in heart failure is unclear, but may occur as a result of pressure overload, for example the excessive demand of afterload on an otherwise normal heart. LVH may also result in impaired cardiac function that is secondary to diastolic dysfunction, subendocardial ischaemia and an inefficient cardiac rhythm due to frequent arrhythmias or even atrial fibrillation. A final mechanism is the association with coronary artery disease, which may result in cardiac ischaemia (with ventricular impairment or 'hibernation') or myocardial infarction (Figure 4.3).

Antihypertensive drugs and LVH

It should be emphasized that LVH is preventable with the use of antihypertensive therapy and improved control of hypertension. In fact, almost every antihypertensive drug is capable of reducing cardiac mass and reversing LVH if therapy is maintained for long enough. The reduction in left ventricular mass also correlates with the reduction in mean arterial pressure.

Not all antihypertensive drugs result in the regression of LVH in a similar fashion. For example, angiotensin-converting enzyme (ACE)

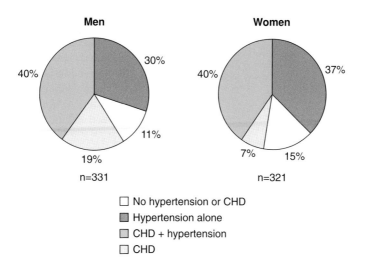

Figure 4.3
Prevalence of coronary heart disease and hypertension in chronic heart failure as seen in the Framingham Heart Study. CHD, coronary heart disease.

inhibitors appear more effective in the regression of LVH than beta-blockers and diuretics (Figure 4.4). By contrast, directly acting vasodilators, such as minoxidil and hydralazine, have little impact on LVH. The effects of left ventricular mass reduction often parallel the reduction in BP as a result of treatment. There is also evidence that cardiac arrhythmias, myocardial ischaemia and impaired ventricular filling diminish in parallel to the reduction in left ventricular mass and the regression of LVH. In the Framingham study, for example, patients with a reduction in LVH showed a decrease of at least 25% in cardiovascular mortality over four years, the effect being most beneficial in men.

In the recent Losartan Intervention For Endpoint reduction in hypertension (LIFE) trial in 'high risk' patients with essential hypertension and ECG evidence LVH, the primary composite endpoint was reduced by 13% with the angiotensin receptor blocker losartan compared to atenolol, and was virtually the result of a

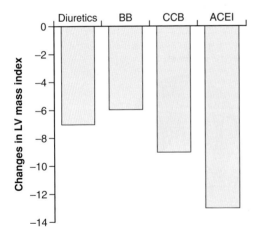

Figure 4.4
Reversal of left ventricular hypertrophy in essential hypertension – meta-analysis data showing changes in left ventricular mass index with different classes of antihypertensive agent. BB, beta-blockers; CCB, calcium channel blockers; ACEI, angiotensin-converting enzyme inhibitors. (Adapted from Schmeider et al. JAMA 1996; **275**: 1507–13.)

25% stroke reduction by losartan. In addition, there was a 25% reduction in cases of new diabetes in patients treated with losartan compared with atenolol.

> Not all antihypertensive drugs operate in the same way to reduce LVH; for example, ACE inhibitors appear to be more effective than beta-blockers and diuretics, while directly acting vasodilators have little impact

Heart failure

Convincing evidence from prospective epidemiological studies suggests that heart failure may be caused by high BP and can be prevented by its control. For example, the Framingham study suggested that high BP was the principal cause of heart failure; subjects with BP >160/95 mmHg had a six-fold higher incidence of heart failure than those with BP <140/90 mmHg. Heart failure has a poor long-term prognosis, and New York Heart Association (NYHA) Grade IV heart failure has a worse prognosis than some cancers, with a one year mortality of >50%. Heart failure in association with untreated hypertension over many years can slowly be replaced by 'normal' BP as the left ventricular muscle progressively fails.

Hypertension is associated with structural changes in the heart that result in increased passive stiffness and impaired diastolic relaxation. This compromises cardiac filling during diastole and reduces cardiac output, resulting in heart failure. Conventional belief suggests that as a result of reduced diastolic filling, left ventricular filling becomes more dependent on heart rate and atrial contribution. Thus, during tachycardia or atrial fibrillation, which reduces diastolic filling time and atrial contribution, stroke volume may be significantly reduced, with consequent increase in end-diastolic pressure and pulmonary oedema. However, rate-lowering drugs such as beta-blockers have not been tested in large clinical trials in patients with heart failure and normal left ventricular ejection fraction.

Other contributory factors include exercise-induced subendocardial ischaemia, which can produce 'exaggerated' impairment of diastolic relaxation of the hypertrophied myocardium, and finally, hypertension in association with renal artery stenosis can cause 'flash' pulmonary oedema, which can be corrected by treatment of the renal artery stenosis.

Large vessel arterial disease

Peripheral vascular disease (PVD) is associated with a high cardiovascular morbidity and mortality. Intermittent claudication is the most common symptomatic manifestation of PVD, but is also an important predictor of cardiovascular death, increasing it three-fold, and increasing all-cause mortality by two to five times.

Hypertension is a common and important risk factor for vascular disorders, including PVD. About 2–5% of hypertensive patients have intermittent claudication at presentation and the prevalence increases with age. Similarly, 35–55% of patients with PVD at presentation also have hypertension. Patients who suffer from hypertension with PVD have a greatly increased risk of myocardial infarction and stroke. Many patients with PVD also have renal artery stenosis, which may contribute to their hypertension. Unless specifically investigated for, this often remains undiagnosed (Figure 4.5).

> The most common symptom of PVD is intermittent claudication, and it also increases the chances of cardiovascular death three-fold

Hypertension is also a major risk factor for aneurysmal dilation of the aorta (thoracic and abdominal). High pulsatile wave stress and atheromatous disease can lead to dissection of the aorta, which carries a high short-term mortality. Extracranial carotid artery disease is also more common in hypertensive patients and is one of the mechanisms by which hypertension leads to the increased risk of stroke.

Despite these well-recognized associations, none of the large antihypertensive treatment trials have adequately studied the benefit of BP reduction on the incidence of PVD and aortic aneurysms. There is an obvious need for such outcome studies to correlate the effect of BP reduction on the incidence of these arterial diseases, especially since the two conditions are commonly encountered together, but the association is often neglected.

> The majority of aortic aneurysms occur in patients with hypertension, where high pulsatile wave stress and atheromatous disease can result in dissection of the aorta

Kidney and renal failure

Renal dysfunction is often found in hypertensive patients and malignant hypertension frequently leads to progressive renal failure. There is some controversy as to whether or not mild-to-moderate essential hypertension leads to renal failure. It may be that patients who develop renal failure in fact have hypertension secondary to renal disease, rather than vice-versa.

In the Renfrew community project, individuals with raised BP had a higher frequency of ECG evidence of left ventricular enlargement assessed by the Minnesota code and slightly larger cardiothoracic ratios on chest X-ray. In

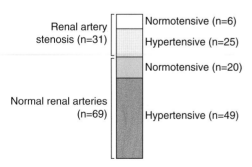

Figure 4.5
Renal artery stenosis in peripheral vascular disease.
(Adapted from Wachtell *et al. J Hum Hypertens* 1996; **10**: 83–5.)

sharp contrast, serum creatinine as an index of renal damage did not differ when comparing hypertensive patients to normotensive patients. If serum creatinine is an index of hypertensive target organ damage as LVH is, then higher serum creatinine levels would be expected in hypertensive patients. Thus the relationship between hypertension and the kidney is qualitatively rather than quantitatively different from the link between hypertension and cardiac or cerebral damage.

Proteinuria

In hypertensive patients, the presence of proteinuria is prognostically important and associated with a roughly two-fold increase in cardiovascular mortality (Figure 4.6). Microproteinuria has been considered to be evidence of early BP-induced kidney damage. Relationships have been found between microproteinuria and the left ventricular mass on echocardiography.

In the INTERSALT (International Study of Salt and Blood Pressure) project, no relationship was found between the height of the systolic or

diastolic BP and the amount of protein in urine. This may be related to the large number of non-BP related causes of proteinuria (non-specific), including fever, heart failure, changes in posture, vigorous exercise and trauma.

There are no reported cases of benign essential hypertensive patients with normal serum creatinine levels and no proteinuria who subsequently went on to develop renal failure. This is in sharp contrast to the relationship between hypertension and its cardiovascular and cerebral complications where uncomplicated benign hypertension frequently leads to the development of heart attacks or strokes. These data strongly suggest that only those patients with primary renal disease will progress to develop end-stage renal failure (Figure 4.7).

Possible mechanisms of renal damage in hypertension

Several hormones, some of which have a renal origin, are involved in the maintenance of BP, renal blood flow and renal function. Most of these mechanisms explain why kidney diseases

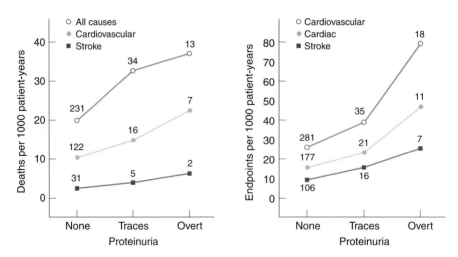

Figure 4.6
The left panel shows age- and gender-adjusted death rates according to the level of proteinuria. The right panel shows the age- and gender-adjusted fatal and non-fatal event rates according to the level of proteinuria. (From De Leeuw *et al.* Prognostic significance of renal function in elderly patients with isolated systolic hypertension: results from the Syst-Eur trial. *J Am Soc Nephrol* 2002; **13**: 2213–22.)

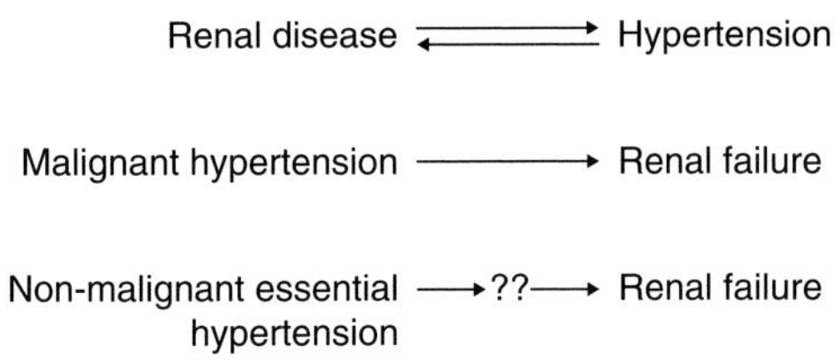

Renal disease ⇄ Hypertension

Malignant hypertension ⟶ Renal failure

Non-malignant essential ⟶??⟶ Renal failure
　　　　　hypertension

Figure 4.7
Hypertension and the kidney – the development of end-stage renal failure.

cause raised BP rather than vice versa. Some patients with hypertension-induced atheromatous disease of their renal arteries might be expected to develop renal impairment but that is not due to intrinsic kidney damage.

Other possible mechanisms include effects of cardiovascular drugs, such as a reduction of cardiac output and renal blood flow due to beta-blockade and a reduction of renal plasma flow in patients treated with ACE inhibitors while in a state of intravascular volume depletion. The vast majority of these patients with benign essential hypertension will not develop any renal damage whether they are treated or untreated.

> Several hormones help maintain BP, renal blood flow and renal functions, and most explain why kidney diseases cause raised BP rather than vice versa

Evidence from treatment trials

Among hypertensive patients, renal damage is rare compared to heart attacks and strokes, and the number of renal events encountered in the randomized trials of treatment is very small. There is a definite lack of difference in renal endpoints in treated versus untreated hypertensive patients, with a tiny number of cases developing renal impairment.

Participants in the MRC trial of mild hypertension (including a cohort from Renfrew) had their serum urea levels measured at

baseline and were restudied after three years; there was no difference at the outset between those patients who were randomized either to placebo, propranolol, or bendrofluazide treatment (Figure 4.8). A tendency to develop a rise in serum creatinine has been noted in African Americans with hypertension. However, it was striking that the relationship between BP at screening and subsequent renal impairment was very weak compared with the close relationship between BP and the subsequent development of heart attack and strokes.

In a meta-analysis of 10 trials involving 26,521 individuals, Hsu found that among patients enrolled into clinical trials with non-malignant hypertension and without renal dysfunction at baseline, treated patients did not have a lower risk of renal dysfunction. Therefore, this meta-analysis questions the link between benign essential hypertension and renal failure in patients without renal disease.

In contrast, the benefit of blood pressure lowering in ameliorating the progression of renal disease is well demonstrated. A meta-analysis of patients with chronic renal disease and albuminuria suggests better outcomes with systolic blood pressures of less than 130 mmHg and indeed, analysis of the Modification of Diet in Renal Disease study suggests that patients with proteinuria (>1 g/24 hours) may benefit from reduction of blood pressure to less than 125/75 mmHg. Hence, a blood pressure goal of 130/80 mmHg for patients with renal disease is recommended by international guidelines.

> Limited evidence exists that controlling BP in non-malignant essential hypertension influenced renal function in patients without renal disease. However, blood pressure reduction in patients *with* renal disease retards the progression of renal dysfunction

Retinopathy

Hypertension leads to vascular changes in the eye, referred to as hypertensive retinopathy.

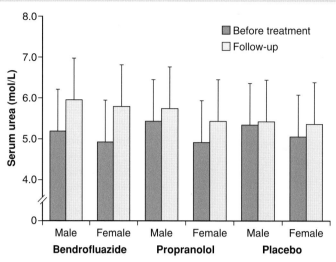

Figure 4.8
Changes in blood urea levels over five years. Data are from the Medical Research Council (MRC) trial. (Adapted from MRC Working Party on Mild Hypertension. *Br Med J* 1986; **293**: 988–92.)

These changes have been classified by Keith, Wagener and Barker into four grades, which correlate with prognosis (Tables 4.7 and 4.8). Malignant hypertension, the most severe form, is clinically defined as raised BP in association with bilateral retinal flame-shaped haemorrhages, and/or cotton wool spots and/or hard exudates, with or without papilloedema.

Table 4.7
The Keith, Wagener, Barker classification

Grade I	Grade II	Grade III	Grade IV
• Benign hypertension	• More marked hypertensive retinopathy	• Mild angiospastic retinopathy	• Malignant hypertension
• Mild narrowing or sclerosis of the retinal arterioles	• Moderate to marked sclerosis of the retinal arterioles	• Retinal oedema, cotton-wool spots and haemorrhages	• All the features in Grades I–III plus optic disc oedema
• No symptoms	• Exaggerated arterial light reflex	• Sclerosis and spastic lesions of retinal arterioles	• Cardiac and renal functions may be impaired
• Good general health	• Venous compression at arteriovenous crossings	• Blood pressure often high and sustained	• Reduced survival
	• Blood pressure higher and more sustained than Group 1	• (Symptomatic)	
	• (Asymptomatic)		
	• Good general health		

Table 4.8

Keith, Wagener, Barker classification – patient survival (Adapted from Keith NM, Wagener HP, Barker NW. Some different types of essential hypertension: their course and prognosis. *Am J Med Sci* 1939; **196**: 332–43)

Years follow-up	Patient survival (%)			
	Grade I	Grade II	Grade III	Grade IV
1	90	88	65	21
3	70	62	22	6
5	70	54	20	1

Further reading

Dahlof B, Pennert K, Hansson L. Reversal of left ventricular hypertrophy in hypertensive patients: a meta-analysis of 109 treatment studies. *Am J Hypertens* 1992; **5**: 95–110.

Dahlof B, Devereux RB, Kjeldsen SE, *et al*. Cardiovascular morbidity and mortality in the Losartan Intervention For Endpoint reduction in hypertension study (LIFE): a randomized trial against atenolol. *Lancet* 2002; **359**: 995–1003.

Levy D, Anderson KM, Savage DD, *et al*. Echocardiographically detected left ventricular hypertrophy: prevalence and risk factors: the Framingham Heart Study. *Ann Intern Med* 1988; **108**: 7–13.

Lip GYH, Felmeden DC, Li-Saw-Hee FL, *et al*. Hypertensive heart disease: a complex syndrome or a hypertensive 'cardiomyopathy'? *Eur Heart J* 2000; **21**: 1653–65.

Rigaud AS, Seux ML, Staessen JA, *et al*. Cerebral complications of hypertension. *J Hum Hypertens* 2000; **14**: 605–16.

Schmieder RE, Messerli FH. Hypertension and the heart. *J Hum Hypertens* 2000; **14**: 597–604.

Schmieder RE, Martus P, Klingbeil A. Reversal of left ventricular hypertrophy in essential hypertension: a meta-analysis of randomized double-blind studies. *JAMA* 1996; **275**: 1507–13.

Schmieder RE, Schlaich MP, Klingbeil AU, *et al*. Update on reversal of left ventricular hypertrophy in essential hypertension (a meta-analysis of all randomized double-blind studies until December 1996). *Nephrol Dial Transplant* 1998; **13**: 564–9.

5. Clinical assessment

Clinical assessment
Investigation of all patients with hypertension
Investigation for secondary causes of hypertension

Clinical assessment

The assessment of the hypertensive patient should include (Table 5.1): confirmation of the diagnosis, assessment of the patient for the underlying cause(s) and target organ damage, identification of concomitant cardiovascular risk factors (to assess overall CVD risk) and identification of compelling indications and contraindications.

The most important aspect of the management of a patient presenting with high blood pressure (BP) is to confirm the diagnosis of hypertension. Multiple measurements of BP over a period of time may show that BP levels fall over time so that a significant number of

Table 5.1
Assessment of hypertensive patients

- Causes of hypertension, e.g. renal disease, endocrine causes
- Contributory factors, e.g. obesity, salt intake, excess alcohol intake
- Complications of hypertension, e.g. previous stroke, left ventricular hypertrophy
- Cardiovascular risk factors, e.g. smoking, family history
- Contraindications to specific drugs, e.g. asthma (beta-blockers), gout (thiazides)

patients can no longer be regarded as hypertensive. Some patients develop high BP in relation to hospital or clinical attendance, the so-called 'white-coat' effect. Patients with white-coat hypertension do not need antihypertensive therapy but do need careful monitoring as these patients may exhibit minor vascular changes and eventually develop overt hypertension in the future. Ambulatory BP monitoring devices have assisted the diagnosis of this condition, with the typical high BPs when the patient is attending the doctor/hospital and virtually normal BPs when the patient is away from the doctor/hospital.

It is a fundamental error to condemn a patient to decades of medication based on only one or two casual BP measurements. Except for hypertensive emergencies or those in high-risk groups (including those exhibiting hypertensive target organ damage), it is good practice to take multiple BP readings over a few months while pursuing non-pharmacological measures before instituting drug therapy.

Multiple measurements of BP are advisable to diagnose hypertension, as a prelude to drug treatments

BP measurement

Despite the important management decisions based upon it, BP measurement in clinical practice is fraught with inaccuracy. Variation in BP readings might occur owing to factors in the patient (biological variation) or problems involving the observer (measurement variation). Frequent observer retraining and a meticulous technique are vital. In an individual patient, BP can vary considerably. BP tends to be highest first thing in the morning and lowest at night, and is higher in cold weather and after consuming caffeine, tobacco or alcohol.

All adults should have BP measured routinely at least every five years until the age of 80 years. Those with high-normal values (135–139/85–89 mmHg) and those who have had high readings at any time previously should have BP re-measured annually. Seated BP recordings are generally sufficient, but standing BP should be measured in elderly or diabetic patients to exclude orthostatic hypotension.

> BP readings should be treated with some caution as a multiplicity of factors can skew the results

Measurement devices

The most accurate device for a non-invasive BP measurement is a well-cared-for mercury manometer; however, mercury is likely to be outlawed in the near future, owing to safety concerns. Aneroid manometers are inaccurate unless regularly calibrated. In the future, it is likely that most BP readings will be made with electronic oscillometric devices, although currently only a few such machines have been carefully validated or certified for clinical use. For example, many devices have failed the British Hypertension Society (BHS) and/or the Association for the Advancement of Medical Instrumentation (AAMI) criteria, although the OMRON HEM 705 CP, OMRON M4 & UA-767 (A&D) have passed. Unfortunately, many devices are marketed without accuracy testing. (For full recommendations of the European Society of Hypertension on blood pressure measuring devices, see O'Brien *et al.* Blood pressure measuring devices: recommendations of the European Society of Hypertension. *Br Med J* 2001; **322**: 531–6, or visit the British Hypertension Society website: www.bhsoc.org for devices that have been tested according to the BHS protocol.)

> Equipment must be regularly calibrated to ensure accuracy of BP measurements

Measurement technique

It is important that the correct sized cuff is used when measuring BP: the width of the air bladder should be equal to about two-thirds the distance from the axilla to the antecubital fossa

and it should encompass at least 80% of the upper arm. The use of too small a cuff will result in an overestimation of the BP. Conversely, oversized cuffs will underestimate the BP.

The patient should be seated in a quiet room with the arm supported at the same level as the heart. The cuff should be inflated to about 20 mmHg above the systolic pressure as indicated by the disappearance of the radial pulse. It should then be deflated at 2–4 mmHg/s and the systolic pressure recorded at the first appearance of the ausculatory sounds, while the diastolic pressure is indicated by the disappearance of the sounds (phase V) (Figure 5.1).

Multiple measurements and monitoring

Management decisions should be made based on readings taken on several occasions over a period of time. An average reading of several measurements taken at separate visits is more accurate than measurements taken at a single visit. In uncomplicated mild hypertension, the average of two readings per visit at monthly intervals over 4–6 months should be used to guide the decision to treat. In more severe hypertension, prolonged observation is not necessary or warranted before treatment. The average BP is only one factor determining cardiovascular risk in uncomplicated mild hypertension. Any formal estimation of CVD risk should heed the consideration of age, sex, smoking habit, diabetes, total cholesterol:high-density lipoprotein (HDL) cholesterol ratio and family history in addition to BP, as described later.

Systolic or diastolic BP?

In practice, systolic BP should be regarded as the more important. Both systolic and diastolic BP are highly correlated, and outcome trials of antihypertensive treatment based on thresholds of diastolic or systolic BP have shown similar reductions in cardiovascular events. Nevertheless, systolic BP is a better predictor of cardiovascular prognosis, correcting for

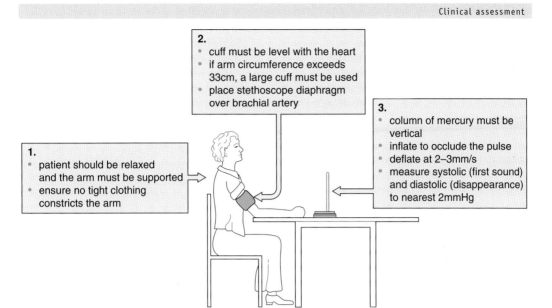

2.
- cuff must be level with the heart
- if arm circumference exceeds 33cm, a large cuff must be used
- place stethoscope diaphragm over brachial artery

3.
- column of mercury must be vertical
- inflate to occlude the pulse
- deflate at 2–3mm/s
- measure systolic (first sound) and diastolic (disappearance) to nearest 2mmHg

1.
- patient should be relaxed and the arm must be supported
- ensure no tight clothing constricts the arm

Figure 5.1
Proper measurement of 'sitting' blood pressure.

underlying diastolic BP. The 2004 British Hypertension Society guidelines recommend a BP treatment target of 140/90 mmHg; this means 140 mmHg systolic or 90 mmHg diastolic in uncomplicated hypertension.

> Systolic BP is a better indicator of cardiovascular risk than diastolic BP

Ambulatory blood pressure monitoring

It is difficult to provide firm guidance on evidence for the use of ambulatory blood pressure monitoring (ABPM) to guide treatment, as all outcome trials in hypertension have been based on surgery or clinic BP, not ABPM. ABPM provides numerous measurements over a short time and reduces variability and measurement error when compared to the average of a limited number of clinic readings. BP by ABPM correlates more closely with evidence of target organ damage.

ABPM may be indicated in the following circumstances:

- when BP shows unusual variability
- in hypertension resistant to drug therapy, defined as BP >150/90 mmHg on a regimen of three or more antihypertensive drugs
- when symptoms suggest the possibility of hypotension
- to diagnose white-coat hypertension.

It is not necessary or feasible to perform ABPM to exclude white-coat hypertension in all hypertensive patients. The term 'white-coat hypertension' has been widely used to describe regular hypertension in the clinic with consistent normotension by ABPM. In these patients, there is a systematic clinic–ABPM difference in the population that is related to the level of clinic BP, and white-coat hypertension is considered to be present only when the clinic–ABPM difference exceeds the population average difference. This white-coat hypertension should be suspected in patients who demonstrate persistently elevated BP yet have little or no evidence of end-organ damage, or who develop symptoms of hypotension on even small doses of antihypertensive drugs.

White-coat hypertension may not need treatment, but should be kept under observation, as many do develop changes in endothelial function, intima thickness, echocardiography that are intermediate between normotensive patients and overt hypertensive patients.

> Ambulatory blood pressure monitoring (ABPM) can be used to provide additional readings for BP, but not to exclude white-coat hypertension

Thus, patients left untreated on the basis of ABPM will need to be followed up, with reassessment of BP and cardiovascular risk at least once-yearly. The annual reassessment may require repeated ABPM measurement.

When interpreting ABPM results, the average daytime BP should be used for treatment decisions, not the average 24-hour BP. Any BP measured by ABPM is systematically lower than surgery or clinic measurements in hypertensive and normotensive people. Thus an ABPM average daytime BP would be expected to be equivalent to 10/5 mmHg lower than the office BP, and both treatment thresholds and targets should be adjusted accordingly.

BP measurement at home

Evidence on the role of self-measurement of BP is less extensive than for ABPM, but many of the same considerations apply. As in ABPM, home blood pressure measurements tend to be systematically lower than clinic BP and BP of ≥135/85 mmHg should be considered the hypertension range.

Patient assessment – beyond blood pressure

The primary purpose of the assessment is to exclude secondary causes (see Table 5.3). Although accounting for fewer than 5% of hypertensive patients, secondary causes of hypertension should be excluded as they are often either correctable or represent serious

underlying disease. Renal and endocrine disease or concomitant medication (such as oestrogen-containing contraceptive pills or non-steroidal anti-inflammatory drugs) account for the majority of the secondary causes of hypertension.

The second purpose is to establish the individual's level of absolute risk. A patient who has had a myocardial infarction is at high risk of further cardiovascular events, and as such will require treatment at lower blood pressure levels. Evidence of hypertensive target organ damage, such as left ventricular hypertrophy (LVH), proteinuria or severe retinopathy are also high-risk features with a lower threshold for blood pressure treatment. Hence, each new patient requires a thorough clinical assessment. A full cardiovascular examination should be accompanied by simple investigations: (i) blood biochemistry for urea and electrolytes, serum creatinine, fasting glucose and cholesterol; (ii) urinalysis for blood, protein and glucose; and (iii) an electrocardiogram (ECG) (Table 5.2).

Thirdly, the individual patient should be assessed for other concomitant conditions or co-morbidities as this will guide antihypertensive therapy. For example, beta-blockers, which are not be recommended for the initial treatment of hypertension, are indicated in patients with heart failure due to

---

Table 5.2
Routine investigations in hypertensive patients (see text for more details)

- Urine strip test, e.g. for protein and blood, which may indicate underlying renal disease
- Serum creatinine and electrolytes, which may raise a clinical suspicion of renal disease, Conn's syndrome, etc.
- Blood glucose, e.g. for associated diabetes
- Total serum:HDL cholesterol, which would allow associated hyperlipidaemia to be treated as part of overall cardiovascular risk prevention
- ECG, e.g. for diagnosis of associated rhythm abnormalities, myocardial infarction, LVH, etc.

left ventricular systolic dysfunction (see Chapter 6). Therefore, antihypertensive therapy may be individualized based on the presence of specific compelling indications or contraindications.

The need for further investigations such as chest X-ray, urine microscopy and culture, renal ultrasound and echocardiography should be individualized. An echocardiogram is valuable to confirm or refute the presence of LVH when the ECG shows 'high' left ventricular voltage without T-wave abnormalities, as is often the case in young patients.

The absolute risk is the probability (range 0 to 1) that an individual will experience the specified outcome during a specified period. The relative risk (RR) is the number of times more likely (RR > 1.0) or less likely (RR < 1.0) an event is to happen in one group compared to another. It is analogous to the odds ratio (OR) when events are rare, and is the ratio of the absolute risk for each group (definition from *Clinical Evidence*).

Investigation of all patients with hypertension

The basic investigations should include blood biochemistry for urea and electrolytes, serum creatinine, fasting glucose and cholesterol, urinalysis for blood, protein and glucose and an ECG.

Urinalysis

Proteinuria and microscopic haematuria might result from renal arteriolar fibrinoid necrosis in patients with malignant hypertension, and also occur in patients with non-malignant hypertension and hypertensive nephrosclerosis. In those cases where proteinuria is present, for a given BP level, the risk of death is roughly doubled. Glycosuria may indicate coincident diabetes mellitus.

Proteinuria and microscopic haematuria may also indicate:

- intrinsic renal disease
  —glomerulonephritis
  —polycystic kidney disease
  —pyelonephritis
- urological malignancy.

Haematology

Anaemia in a hypertensive patient may be due to renal impairment. Polycythaemia may be seen in patients with chronic obstructive airways disease, Cushing's syndrome, alcohol excess and, very rarely, renal carcinoma. Plasma viscosity or erythrocyte sedimentation rate should be measured if there is a suspicion of some underlying vasculitic disease.

Biochemical investigations

Serum sodium concentration may be raised or in the high-normal range in patients with primary hyperaldosteronism (Conn's syndrome). In patients with secondary hyperaldosteronism, as occurs in chronic renal failure, serum sodium concentration can be low or low-normal. Low serum sodium levels are also produced by high doses of diuretics; occasionally profound hyponatraemia may be encountered in combination therapy, such as Moduret (amiloride and hydrochlorothiazide).

Serum potassium concentration is usually low or low-normal in patients with Conn's syndrome, but the most common cause of hypokalaemia is diuretic therapy. Hyperkalaemia may be found in renal failure or with the use of some antihypertensive drugs such as the angiotensin-converting enzyme (ACE) inhibitors or the potassium-sparing diuretics (e.g. spironolactone or amiloride).

> Different serum sodium concentrations indicate different conditions such as Conn's syndrome (high-normal) or secondary hyperaldosteronism (low or low-normal)

Life-threatening hyperkalaemia has been described in patients receiving an ACE inhibitor who then opted to consume a salt substitute (Lo-Salt), which contains potassium chloride instead of sodium chloride. Monitoring of electrolytes is also important with the use of diuretics and ACE inhibitors; in particular, ACE inhibitors and potassium-sparing diuretics should not be used together unless very careful monitoring of serum potassium is undertaken.

Serum urea and creatinine concentrations should be monitored as hypertension may cause renal impairment and renal diseases cause hypertension. A graph plotting the reciprocal of the serum creatinine against time may give an indication of the rate of deterioration of renal function, and hence predict the need for intervention and renal dialysis. Increasingly, laboratories are now reporting estimated glomerular filtration rates, which allows direct assessment of renal function over time. Of note, a rise in serum creatinine early after the initiation of an ACE inhibitor is common. In a review of 12 clinical trials by Bakris and Weir, a rise in serum creatinine of up to 30% that stabilizes within the first two months of ACE inhibitor therapy is associated with long-term preservation of renal function. Based on this study, ACE inhibitors should not be withdrawn in patients with a minor (<30%) rise in serum creatinine.

Primary hyperparathyroidism, which is associated with hypertension, causes a raised serum calcium concentration with a low serum phosphate concentration. As with serum potassium, these results may be affected by the use of diuretic therapy, which modestly raises serum calcium.

Hyperuricaemia is found in about 40% of hypertensive patients, in association with renal impairment. Serum uric acid rises with increased alcohol ingestion or the use of thiazide diuretics. Raised gamma-glutamyl transferase levels strongly suggest an excessive alcohol intake, assuming that other intrinsic liver diseases have been excluded.

Elevated serum cholesterol and triglyceride levels with low high-density lipoprotein (HDL) cholesterol levels are synergistic risk factors that need to be assessed in all hypertensive patients and treated if necessary. They may also be elevated very slightly by the use of some antihypertensive agents, such as the thiazide diuretics and non-selective beta-blockers. Concomitant cardiovascular risk factors are common in patients with hypertension (Figure 5.2) and should be actively sought and treated.

> Two-fifths of hypertensive patients have hyperuricaemia in association with renal impairment

Electrocardiography

The ECG should be a routine investigation in all hypertensive patients, providing a baseline with which later changes may be compared. An ECG may show evidence of underlying ischaemic heart disease and is useful to screen for the presence of LVH. However, a normal ECG does not exclude the presence of LVH and there is a strong case for using echocardiography to more regularly diagnose cardiac enlargement.

The diagnosis of LVH by electrocardiogram has been described previously (see Chapter 4). The presence of LVH provides clear evidence of end-organ damage and a three- to four-fold excess mortality, and indicates the need for aggressive BP control. The prognosis is even worse if the 'strain' pattern of ST inversion is also seen in leads V5 and V6.

> Despite not being able to exclude LVH, ECGs should be used more frequently to diagnose cardiac enlargements

Investigation for secondary causes of hypertension

Secondary causes of hypertension are listed in Table 5.3. These should be considered in selected patient populations (Table 5.4).

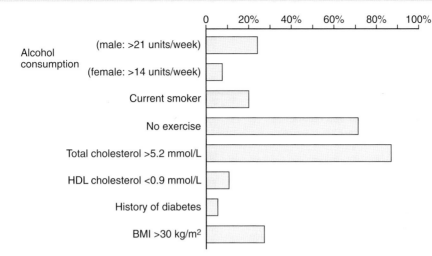

Figure 5.2
Concomitant risk factors in hypertensive patients. HDL, high-density lipoprotein; BMI, body mass index. (Adapted from Poulter *et al. Blood Pressure* 1996; **5:** 209–15.)

Table 5.3
Secondary causes of hypertension

Endocrine:
—Cushing's syndrome
—Conn's syndrome
—phaeochromocytoma
—hyper/hypothyroidism
—acromegaly
—hypercalcaemia
—carcinoid
—exogenous hormones, e.g. contraceptive pill,
  glucocorticoids
Renal:
—glomerulonephritis
—diabetic nephropathy
—polycystic kidney disease
—renal artery stenosis (fibromuscular or
  atherosclerotic)
Coarctation of the aorta
Raised intracranial pressure
Pregnancy-induced hypertension
Alcohol and drug abuse
Acute stress

Table 5.4
Patients who require further investigations

- The young (aged <40 years)
- Those with severe hypertension (diastolic blood pressure >120 mmHg)
- Those with resistant or uncontrolled hypertension
- Those with a suspicion of underlying pathology (i.e. secondary hypertension)

trigger further analyses including urinary microscopy for red and white cell casts to exclude glomerulonephritis and vasculitis. This should prompt referral to specialist services. Similarly, specialist referral should be considered in patients with dipstick proteinuria and urinary protein:creatinine ratio of > 100 mg/mmol. Of note, renal dysfunction in patients with diabetes should not be immediately assumed to represent diabetic nephropathy, especially in the absence of other concomitant microvascular disease (e.g. retinopathy).

Renal disease

Urinalysis and renal ultrasound are crucial for the diagnosis of renal disease. The identification of persistent unexplained haematuria should

Renal ultrasonography is useful in demonstrating renal anatomy, for example, hydronephrosis, abnormal polycystic kidneys, or diminished renal size. A unilateral, smooth, small kidney may indicate renal artery stenosis. In patients with intrinsic renal disease the kidneys may appear 'bright' on ultrasonography. Renal ultrasound may be justified in patients with hypertension and renal bruit, abnormal renal function, severe deterioration in renal function with ACE inhibitors and recurrent hospital admissions with 'flash' pulmonary oedema.

Phaeochromocytoma

Phaeochromocytomas are catecholamine-producing neuroendocrine tumours arising most commonly in the adrenal glands. The prevalence of phaeochromocytoma among patients with hypertension is low (<1%), but the consequences of a missed diagnosis are often fatal. Hence a high index of suspicion is required and should be supported by biochemical testing. Symptoms and signs are usually non-specific and include headaches, flushing, palpitations, sweats and sometimes even postural hypotension.

Twenty-four-hour urine collections for catecholamines and vanillyl mandelic acid (VMA) are traditionally used for the diagnosis of phaeochromocytoma. However, more recent data suggest higher sensitivity with measurement of plasma and urinary metanephrines.

Primary aldosteronism

Primary aldosteronism is characterized by hypertension, suppressed plasma renin activity (PRA) and increased plasma aldosterone concentration (PAC). Conn's syndrome refers to an uncommon subtype of primary aldosteronism due to an underlying aldosterone-secreting adenoma. A more common subtype, however, is idiopathic hyperaldosteronism characterized by bilateral hyperplasia of the zona glomerulosa. Using a high PAC:PRA ratio in the presence of high PAC (values dependent on local laboratories), the prevalence of primary aldosteronism may be as high as 12% of patients referred to a tertiary centre. The

prevalence is higher in patients with more severe hypertension. PAC:PRA ratio should therefore be considered for patients with resistant hypertension.

Cushing's syndrome

Investigations for Cushing's syndrome should be conducted in all patients with a 'cushingoid' appearance (a plethoric round face, hirsutism, central obesity with red abdominal striae, thin skin and easy bruising). In addition, screening for Cushing's syndrome may be considered in obese patients with uncontrolled glucose and hypertension (especially in association with hypokalaemia).

Random cortisol assays can be misleading and should not be routinely performed. Assessment

Table 5.5
Key issues to consider in imaging

Factors to consider:
- intravenous urography is no longer used in the investigation of hypertension
- renal angiography is the gold standard for the diagnosis of renal artery stenosis, although the procedure does carry some risk
- magnetic resonance (MR) renal angiography is replacing renal angiography as the investigation of choice to diagnose renal artery stenosis
- computed tomography (CT) or magnetic resonance imaging (MRI) can be used for the localization of phaeochromocytomas or adrenal tumours causing aldosterone excess, but beware of non-hormone-secreting incidentalomas detected on CT or MRI
- standard renal radioisotope imaging now has little to offer in the investigation of hypertension
- radioisotope imaging may also be useful in the localization of phaeochromocytomas using scans with metaiodo-benzylguanidene (MIBG scan)
- iodo-cholesterol radioisotope imaging has little value in the diagnosis of aldosterone-secreting adrenal adenomas
- echocardiography is primarily of use in the investigation of structural heart disease, including valvular heart disease and left ventricular dysfunction

of the 24-hour urinary free cortisol (multiple 24-hour collections are generally recommended) and overnight dexamethasone (1 mg) suppression test are useful initial biochemical tests. Clinical suspicion or abnormal biochemical tests should prompt specialist referral as the diagnosis poses significant diagnostic challenge. Imaging tests should not be requested without concomitant biochemical evaluation (Table 5.5).

Acromegaly and hyperparathyroidism

Acromegaly may be suspected from the patient's clinical features; it is investigated through glucose tolerance testing, with measurement of growth hormone and insulin-like growth factor-1 (IGF-1) levels, and imaging of the pituitary fossa. Primary hyperparathyroidism is diagnosed by the presence of a normal or raised parathyroid hormone concentration in the presence of a raised serum calcium concentration.

Further reading

JBS 2: Joint British Societies' guidelines on prevention of cardiovascular disease in clinical practice. *Heart* 2005; **91**: 1–52.

O'Brien E, Waeber B, Parati G, *et al*. Blood pressure measuring devices: recommendations of the European Society of Hypertension. *BMJ* 2001; **322**: 531–6.

Seventh Report of the Joint National Committee on Prevention, Detection, Evaluation and Treatment of High Blood Pressure. *Hypertension* 2003; **42**: 1206–52.

Williams B, Poulter NR, Brown MJ, *et al*. Guidelines for management of hypertension: report of the fourth working party of the British Hypertension Society. *J Hum Hypertens* 2004; **18**: 139–85.

Young Jr WF. Primary aldosteronism – changing concepts in diagnosis and treatment. *Endocrinology* 2003; **144**: 2208–23.

6. Treatment

Cardiovascular risk and antihypertensive therapy
Non-pharmacological management
Pharmacological management
Multifactorial interventions to prevent cardiovascular disease
Resistant hypertension
Combination antihypertensive therapy
Clinical guidelines

There is almost a dose–response relationship between increasing stroke and coronary risk with increasing blood pressure (BP), while evidence from clinical trials suggests that BP lowering is associated with a marked reduction in cardiovascular events. Therefore, there is no doubt that patients at high risk of cardiovascular events require aggressive BP lowering.

The current approach to the management of hypertension is to take into account the patient's individual characteristics in terms of concomitant disease and risk factors, as well as social and economic considerations, in deciding on the most appropriate therapy.

> Many factors must be taken into account when deciding on appropriate treatment for a hypertensive patient

This chapter provides an overview of the management of hypertension, predominantly based upon the 2004 British Hypertension Society guidelines. These 2004 guidelines, however, preceded the publication of several landmark clinical trials. More recently, the National Institute of Clinical Excellence (NICE) has taken the data from these clinical trials into consideration and issued a partial update on the previous guidelines.

Cardiovascular risk and antihypertensive therapy

Absolute blood pressure and absolute cardiovascular risk

The individual's blood pressure level, presence of other cardiovascular risk factors (e.g. diabetes and dyslipidaemia) or atherosclerotic vascular disease (e.g. coronary heart disease, stroke or peripheral vascular disease) determines the risk of cardiovascular disease (CVD). The threshold for initiating treatment should reflect these clinical factors.

The British Hypertension Society and Joint British Societies consider the following patient groups at high risk of CVD:

- patients with persistently high blood pressure (≥ 160/100 mmHg)
- cardiovascular complications (e.g. previous stroke or coronary disease)
- target organ damage (e.g. left ventricular hypertrophy (LVH))
- type 1 and type 2 diabetes
- renal dysfunction
- total cholesterol:HDL cholesterol ratio >6 or inherited dyslipidaemia.

Therefore, further risk assessment is not required and antihypertensive treatment should be initiated even for patients with 'mild' hypertension (140–159/90–99 mmHg).

For patients with hypertension without these high-risk features, the decision to start antihypertensive treatment should be guided by further CVD risk assessment. Intuitive estimates of absolute risk are very inaccurate, and while risk estimation is improved when additional risk factors are simply counted, it is significantly more accurate when all major risk factors are counted and weighted using risk functions derived from epidemiological studies, most commonly the Framingham risk function.

> Even mild hypertension must be treated if the patient has additional cardiovascular problems

Risk assessment

The 1999 British Hypertension Society guidelines used the Joint British Societies recommendations on preventing coronary heart diseases (CHD), which included a computer program (the 'Cardiac risk assessor') and a CHD risk chart, both of which are based on the Framingham risk function. The second Joint British Societies guidelines now recommend a move away from CHD risk to the more global CVD risk. The latter includes the risk of stroke (fatal/non-fatal stroke, intracerebral haemorrhage and transient ischaemic attack (TIA), in addition to coronary events). The new CVD charts are also based on the Framingham risk function and specify three levels of 10-year CVD risk: ≥30%, ≥20% and ≤10%, which are equivalent to CHD risk of 23%, 15% and 8% respectively. These three groups are represented by three colour bands on the chart for easy use (see Chapter 2, Table 2.1).

The targeting of antihypertensive treatment at absolute (CVD) risk is underpinned by evidence from meta-analyses of outcome trials. These studies show that the relative risk reduction by antihypertensive treatment is approximately constant, with a 38% reduction in stroke and 16% reduction in coronary events. In patients with mild hypertension, treatment reduces cardiovascular complications by approximately 25%. Treatment of patients at a 10-year CVD risk of ≥ 20% corresponds to a number needed to treat (NNT) for five years of 40 (i.e. treatment of 40 patients for five years to prevent one cardiovascular complication). Assessment of CVD risk also guides the use of aspirin or statins in hypertensive patients. Decisions on treatment at lower levels of CVD risk will be influenced by the patient's attitude

to treatment, and the benefit anticipated from treatment.

It is recommended that all patients with average BP 140–159 or 90–99 mmHg should be offered antihypertensive drug treatment if:

- there is any complication of hypertension or target organ damage, or diabetes
- the 10-year CVD risk is ≥ 20% despite advice on non-pharmacological measures. (Source: British Hypertension Society, 2004)

> Treatment of hypertensive patients can reduce the risk of strokes by 38% and of coronary events by 16%

Monitoring

The British Hypertension Society guidelines recommend that when a decision is reached not to treat a patient with mild hypertension, it is essential to continue observation and monitoring of their BP, at least yearly. Certainly, in about 10–15% of patients, BP levels rise in five years to levels clearly requiring treatment. Age is obviously an important consideration, and risk should be reassessed at yearly intervals. Non-pharmacological measures should be encouraged, to lower BP and cardiovascular risk.

> Yearly monitoring of BP is essential, even in mildly hypertensive patients

Thresholds for intervention

Antihypertensive therapy should be started as follows:

- Accelerated (malignant) hypertension (papilloedema, fundal haemorrhages and exudates) or impending cardiovascular complications: admit for immediate treatment.
- BP ≥ 220/120 mmHg: treat immediately.
- BP 200–219/110–119 mmHg: confirm over 1–2 weeks, then treat.

- BP 160–199/100–109 mmHg:
  —cardiovascular complications/target organ damage or diabetes (type 1 or 2) present: confirm over 3–4 weeks, then treat
  —cardiovascular complications/target organ damage or diabetes (type 1 or 2) absent: non-pharmacological advice, re-measure weekly and treat if BP persists at these levels over 4–12 weeks.
- BP 140–159/90–99 mmHg:
  —cardiovascular complications/target organ damage or diabetes (type 1 or 2) present: confirm and treat
  —cardiovascular complications/target organ damage or diabetes (type 1 or 2) absent: non-pharmacological advice, re-measure at monthly intervals.
- If mild hypertension persists, estimate 10-year CVD risk formally using the second Joint British Societies CVD risk chart. Treat if the estimated 10-year CVD risk ≥ 20%. (Source: British Hypertension Society, 2004)

Non-pharmacological management

Before a patient is commenced on antihypertensive medication, it is always appropriate to attempt non-pharmacological measures to lower BP, except in a few high-risk cases where they should be applied in parallel. Certainly, non-pharmacological measures can be synergistic with drugs, e.g. salt restriction and the use of diuretics. Elderly and Afro-Caribbean patients are examples where such an approach may be useful. Benefits of non-pharmacological methods are listed in Table 6.1.

> Non-pharmacological methods of lowering BP should be attempted first

A number of lifestyle modifications (e.g. weight reduction, salt and alcohol restriction and regular exercise) may produce significant falls in BP and can also improve other cardiovascular risk factors.

Table 6.1
Benefits of non-pharmacological methods to treat hypertension

- Lowers blood pressure as much as drug monotherapy
- Reduces the need for drug therapy
- Enhances the antihypertensive effect of drugs
- Reduces the need for multiple drug regimens
- Favourably influences overall cardiovascular risk

The epidemiologists would advocate that a population strategy could potentially prevent the rise in BP with age, reduce the prevalence of hypertension and need for drug therapy, and reduce overall cardiovascular risk in a population. The public health initiatives for such a strategy include a diet that is:

- high in fruit and vegetables
- high in legumes and whole grains
- high in fat-free and low-fat dairy products, poultry, fish, shellfish and meat products
- high in all essential nutrients
- reduced in salt
- reduced in total fat, saturated fat and cholesterol
- low in alcohol (with no more than 2–3 units per day)
- calorie-controlled to prevent or correct obesity.

In individual patients, changes in diet and lifestyle do lower BP and may also reduce cardiovascular risk.

> Sensible diet leads to lower blood pressure

Conversely, failure to adopt these measures may attenuate the response to antihypertensive drugs. Clear verbal and written advice should be provided for all hypertensive patients and also for those with high-normal BP or a strong family history.

The British Hypertension Society guidelines suggest that in patients with mild hypertension but no cardiovascular complications or target organ damage, the response to these measures may be observed up to 6 months. In patients with severe hypertension, non-pharmacological measures should also be instituted in parallel with drug treatment, and should be backed up by simple written information. Effective implementation of these non-pharmacological measures requires enthusiasm, knowledge, patience and considerable time spent with patients and other family members. A summary of the recommendations in the British Hypertension Society guidelines is as follows:

Measures that lower BP:

- weight reduction
- reduced salt intake
- reduced alcohol consumption
- physical exercise
- increased fruit and vegetable consumption
- reduced total fat and saturated fat intake.

Measures to reduce cardiovascular risk:

- stop smoking
- replace saturated fat with polyunsaturated and monounsaturated fats
- increase oily fish consumption
- reduce total fat intake.

Weight reduction

Weight reduction results in BP reduction of about 2.5/1.5 mmHg for each kilogram lost and, in addition, could also improve lipid profile and insulin resistance. Pharmacological intervention to improve weight loss is generally only recommended as part of an overall treatment plan in patients with obesity with cardiovascular risk factors, including hypertension. Orlistat is preferable to sibutramine as the latter increases blood pressure and is not recommended for patients with hypertension. Orlistat, however, is associated with significant gastrointestinal effects intrinsic to its mechanism of action (orlistat reduces absorption of fat molecules).

More recently, the novel endocannabinoid receptor CB1 antagonist rimonabant has been shown to enhance weight loss (again, as part of an overall treatment plan) compared to placebo. This is associated with significant improvement in risk factor profile, including blood pressure lowering, improvement in dyslipidaemia and glycaemic control. Rimonabant has also been shown to improve smoking cessation rates although it is currently only licensed for the treatment of obesity.

Salt reduction

Salt reduction from a daily average of 10 g to 5 g (5 g ≈1 teaspoon) can lower average BP by about 5/3 mmHg, and is particularly effective in the elderly and those with higher initial BP levels. In most people eating a western diet, dietary sodium intake is grossly in excess of that required for good health. Hypertensive patients should thus be advised to avoid adding salt to cooking or at the table. Vast quantities of salt are contained in processed foods such as bread (one slice contains 0.5 g), some breakfast cereals and flavour enhancers such as stock cubes or manufactured sauces, and should be avoided. Salt substitutes containing potassium chloride may be beneficial, but can cause life-threatening hyperkalaemia when combined with angiotensin-converting enzyme (ACE) inhibitors or potassium-sparing diuretics. Almost certainly, salt restriction may be useful in combination with antihypertensive therapy.

Alcohol consumption

Alcohol intake should generally be limited to <21 units per week. Hypertensive patients should be advised to limit their alcohol intake to 21 units per week for men and 14 units per week for women. Chronic excessive alcohol intake is associated with hypertension as well as other adverse cardiac effects, e.g. atrial fibrillation or alcoholic cardiomyopathy. Binge drinking is associated with an increased risk of stroke. Consumption of smaller amounts of alcohol, up to the recommended limit, may protect against CHD and should not be discouraged.

Regular exercise

Exercise on a regular basis should be encouraged, and the type of exercise should be 'regular and dynamic' (e.g. brisk walking) rather than 'isometric' (e.g. weight training). For example, three vigorous training sessions per week may be appropriate for fit younger patients, or brisk walking for 20 minutes each day for older patients. Indeed, 30–45 minutes of modest aerobic exercise, such as a brisk walk or a swim, three times a week would produce a modest fall in BP.

Fruit and vegetable consumption

Increased fruit and vegetable consumption, from two to seven portions daily, lowers BP in hypertensive patients by 7/3 mmHg. This effect may be a consequence of increased potassium intake. When this is done in combination with an increase in low-fat dairy products and a reduction of saturated and total fat, BP falls may be larger, averaging 11/6 mmHg in hypertensive patients and 4/2 mmHg in those with high-normal BP.

Smoking cessation

Cigarette smoking substantially increases cardiovascular risk, and is a greater threat than mild hypertension. Hypertensive patients who smoke should be given advice and help to stop smoking. The use of nicotine replacement therapies approximately doubles the smoking cessation rate.

Saturated fat consumption

Serum cholesterol is additive to the risk of CVD. All patients should be advised to reduce saturated fat and cholesterol intake and to use polyunsaturated and monounsaturated fats instead. Most diet changes will only reduce serum cholesterol by an average of 6%, and there are great difficulties in implementing and sustaining these measures. Thus, many will need aspirin and statin treatment in addition to non-pharmacological measures.

Pharmacological management

It is now well established that hypertension confers an increased risk of heart attacks and strokes, and treatment of high BP reduces this risk. There is a wide variety of antihypertensive agents, although most can be classified into one of five major classes. Each of these drug classes has merits and disadvantages, as well as ancillary properties that influence the choice for a particular patient. In addition, many patients require more than one agent to control their BP, so the choice of sensible combination therapy with appropriate synergistic effects of the drugs becomes important.

Choice of drug

The ideal drug should have a predictable dose–response curve, as well as an acceptable, recognized side-effect profile. The issue of 24-hour control has also increasingly been recognized as important. BP tends to be highest first thing in the morning and this is when the majority of cardiac events occur. A short-acting drug, even if taken the evening before, may have worn off by the time the patient rises in the morning, whereas a drug with a longer half-life will still be protecting the patient.

A drug with a long half-life also has the advantage of only being taken once daily which improves compliance, especially given that up to 30% of patients miss at least one dose weekly. For example, the ACE inhibitor trandolapril maintains >50% of its activity 48 hours after the last dose.

As the purpose of treating hypertension is to reduce the incidence of hypertensive complications, particularly CHD and stroke, the ideal drug should have trial evidence to show that it achieves these ends as well as simply lowering BP.

For each major class of antihypertensive drug there are indications and contraindications for use in specific patient groups. When none of the special considerations apply, the least expensive drug with the most supportive trial evidence – a low dose of a thiazide diuretic – should be preferred.

> The ideal drug is a once-daily drug giving 24-hour control, prolonging protection and reducing the risk of patients missing a dose

Clinical studies

Recent long-term double-blind studies have compared the major classes of antihypertensive drugs (thiazides, beta-blockers, calcium antagonists, ACE inhibitors and alpha-blockers) and showed no consistent or important differences as regards antihypertensive efficacy, side-effects or quality of life.

Overall, these outcome trials have shown significant reductions in stroke by 38%, in coronary events by 16% (less than the 20–25% reduction that is predicted from epidemiological observations) and in cardiovascular mortality by 21%. However, there were differences in the average response between drug classes that were linked to age and ethnic group. The absolute benefit from treatment is smaller in women than men, but this is compatible with their lower cardiovascular risk.

Until recently, there were few trials that compared different classes of drugs directly with regard to reduction in cardiovascular events. However, differences between regimens based on different drug classes are now becoming evident.

> Recent clinical trials suggest differences between classes of drugs in reducing cardiovascular events

Thiazide diuretics

Thiazide diuretics act to reduce the reabsorption of sodium and chloride in the early part of the distal convoluted tubule of the kidney. This results in the delivery of increased amounts of sodium to the distal tubule where some of it is exchanged for potassium. The net result is increased excretion of sodium, potassium and water. Circulating volume is diminished, reducing preload on the heart and thereby lowering cardiac output and BP. With long-term therapy, autoregulation by the body's compensatory mechanisms results in vasodilatation, reduction of peripheral vascular resistance and return of the cardiac output to normal. Thiazides may also have some direct vasodilatory properties. Newer thiazide-like agents such as indapamide may have ancillary direct effect on the myocardium, resulting in regression of LVH.

Thiazides are rapidly absorbed orally and produce a prolonged diuresis. Loop diuretics exert their effects on the loop of Henle and when combined with thiazide diuretics, especially metolazone may result in profound diuresis due to 'sequential nephron blockade'. Hence, combined use of different diuretics requires greater monitoring of patients.

There is no reason not to start treatment with a diuretic in the uncomplicated hypertensive and in fact many clinicians would advocate their use. While there is a flat dose–response curve in terms of blood pressure lowering effect, the side-effect profile is significantly increased at higher doses and low doses should, therefore, be used. Maximal response is obtained at relatively low doses, such as 12.5 mg hydrochlorothiazide or 1.25–2.5 mg bendroflumethiazide. Further increases in dose simply increase side-effects with little further effect on BP. Thus, higher doses of thiazide diuretics (bendroflumethiazide >2.5 mg or hydrochlorothiazide >25 mg daily) are unnecessary and should not be used. On the whole, standard doses of thiazides lower BP as much as other first-line antihypertensives. In some patient groups, e.g. Afro-Caribbean patients and elderly patients, thiazides are particularly effective. Conversely, however, they tend to be less effective in younger Caucasian patients.

There is little to choose between the various thiazides, although it seems prudent to use agents such as hydrochlorothiazide and bendroflumethiazide, which have been proven to be effective at low doses in clinical trials. Newer agents, such as indapamide, have fewer metabolic side-effects and as mentioned above, may even regress hypertensive LVH on echocardiography.

> Use of thiazides leads to increased excretion of sodium, potassium and water, and lowers cardiac output and BP

Clinical studies of thiazide diuretics

Thiazides are one of the classes of antihypertensives that have been extensively tested in large clinical trials. In early trials, thiazides reduced the incidence of stroke by the 40% expected from epidemiological studies, although the reduction in CHD was disappointing. This was perhaps due to the adverse metabolic effects of the large doses used. More recent trials using lower doses have demonstrated impressive reductions in both strokes and heart disease, especially in the elderly. The reduction in coronary events in trials based on low-dose thiazides has been significantly larger, at 28%, than those in trials of regimens based on high-dose thiazide or beta-blocker. Low-dose thiazide-based regimens also significantly reduced cardiovascular and all-cause mortality. The larger benefit on coronary events observed in these trials using low-dose thiazides is not necessarily related to the dose of thiazide as such. It may be related to differences in age, to more effective potassium conservation in these trials or to chance.

In the ALLHAT study involving over 40,000 patients with hypertension, there was no difference in the primary endpoint or mortality between thiazide diuretics, ACE inhibitor and calcium channel blocker.

In the LIVE study, the thiazide-like agent indapamide SR 1.5 mg was compared to enalapril 20 mg over a period of one year. Both agents significantly reduced BP, but only

indapamide SR had a significant effect on left ventricular mass, reducing it by 5.8% compared to 1.9% with enalapril (Figure 6.1). The addition of indapamide to the ACE inhibitor perindopril was also associated with significant reductions in recurrent strokes in the PROGRESS study (among patients with previous stroke or TIA).

Hence, thiazide diuretics are effective antihypertensive agents and may be used as first-line treatment in most patients, especially in patients with low renin state (see later).

Adverse effects

Predictably, thiazide diuretics cause hypokalaemia due to renal potassium wasting. Hypokalaemia may result in ventricular arrhythmias and cause adverse drug effects in patients on digoxin or drugs that prolong the QT interval on the ECG (e.g. Class I anti-arrhythmics, tricyclic antidepressants, antihistamines).

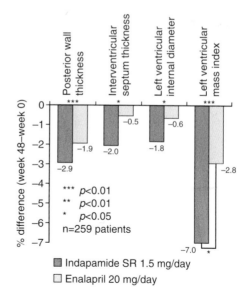

Figure 6.1
Beneficial effects of thiazide on cardiac dimensions; not only do they reduce blood pressure but they can also have a significant effect on left ventricular mass. (Adapted from Gosse *et al. J Hypertens* 2000; **18:** 1465–75.)

Acute gout is another common side-effect of thiazides even when taken in low doses. Hyperuricaemia can be present in about 30% of hypertensives, but is a poor predictor of acute gout.

Thiazide diuretics can increase serum LDL-cholesterol and triglyceride levels, impair glucose tolerance and exacerbate insulin resistance. However, the provocation of overt diabetes is uncommon. Indeed, these adverse metabolic complications are less likely to be a problem at the (low) doses recommended. In hyperlipidaemic and diabetic hypertensive patients, the benefits gained from blood pressure lowering and consequent reduction in cardiovascular risk with low-dose diuretics outweigh these potential metabolic changes. Hence, these metabolic effects should not preclude their use in patients with hypertension.

Rarer side-effects include nausea, headache, rashes, photosensitivity and blood dyscrasias.

> Thiazides can cause metabolic side-effects but are unlikely to pose such problems at low doses

Other diuretics

Loop diuretics act on the ascending limb of the loop of Henle to inhibit the reabsorption of chloride, sodium and potassium. They produce a brisk but short-lived diuresis and are therefore *unsuitable as first-line agents for hypertension* as they lack 24-hour control. They do, however, have a role in those with impaired renal function in whom thiazides are ineffective, and in patients with hypertension resistant to multiple drug therapy who are often fluid overloaded. Furthermore, they may be synergistic with agents such as the ACE inhibitors.

Potassium-sparing diuretics, such as amiloride and triamterene, produce little reduction in BP. They may be useful in combination with other

diuretics to prevent hypokalaemia. Spironolactone is a specific aldosterone antagonist, with a particular role in primary hyperaldosteronism or Conn's syndrome. Eplerenone is also an aldosterone antagonist, albeit with lower receptor affinity (less potent) but higher specificity (fewer anti-androgenic side-effects). The use of aldosterone antagonists is likely to increase with growing recognition of primary aldosteronism (see Chapter 5, 'Primary aldosteronism'). Spironolactone and eplerenone have prognostic benefit in patients with heart failure due to left ventricular systolic dysfunction (RALES study), and heart failure post-myocardial infarction (EPHESUS study) respectively. Serum potassium, however, should be monitored, especially if used in conjunction with ACE inhibitors and in patients with renal failure.

Beta-adrenergic receptor blockers

Beta-adrenergic receptor blockers act by blocking the action of noradrenaline (norepinephrine) at beta-adrenoreceptors throughout the circulatory system and elsewhere. As a class, beta-blockers are heterogeneous with varying selectivity for beta$_1$-adrenoreceptors, their intrinsic sympathomimetic activity and other associated effects on alpha-adrenoreceptors, antioxidative and nitric oxide modulating effects. Their major effect is to slow the heart rate and reduce the force of contraction of the heart. Beta-blockers also cause some reduction in renin release and central sympathetic tone.

The beta$_1$-receptor blockers or cardioselective agents, such as atenolol, have relatively less action on beta$_2$-adrenoreceptors in the bronchi and peripheral vessels, when compared to a non-selective agent such as propranolol. This reduces (but does not totally abolish) beta$_2$-receptor-mediated side-effects. Some beta-blockers, such as pindolol, have intrinsic sympathomimetic activity where they stimulate beta-adrenoreceptors when the background sympathetic nervous activity is low, and block beta-adrenoreceptors when background sympathetic nervous activity is high. They cause less bradycardia and fewer problems with cold extremities than conventional beta-blockers, but in practice are not regularly used in the treatment of hypertension. Labetalol and carvedilol have both alpha-blocking and beta$_1$-blocking properties, leading to a reduction in peripheral vascular resistance as well as slowing the heart rate. They have the disadvantage of possessing the side-effects of both classes of drug. In addition to its beta$_1$-blocking properties, carvedilol also has antioxidant effects, which may have advantages in reducing endothelial damage and lowering levels of highly atherogenic oxidized LDL-cholesterol.

Nebivolol is a highly selective antagonist of the beta$_1$-receptor with vasodilatory properties associated with modulation of nitric oxide production. Studies suggest greater short-term (three months) BP lowering compared to other beta-blockers (metoprolol), ACE inhibitor (enalapril) and calcium channel blocker (nifedipine), with low incidence of beta-blocker-related side-effects.

Efficacy of beta-blockers

Beta-blockers have been used as first-line antihypertensive agents for many years, but recent data are now challenging this practice. Beta-blockers were previously noted to be less effective in the elderly and in Afro-Caribbean patients. Recent meta-analysis suggests that beta-blockers may be ineffective in reducing the risk of myocardial infarction compared to placebo and reduced the risk of stroke by only about half of that expected from previous studies (19% compared to 38%). The efficacy of atenolol in particular has been called into question, with a meta-analysis suggesting higher mortality with atenolol compared to other antihypertensive agents, despite similar reductions in blood pressure. The combination of bendroflumethiazide and atenolol was also shown to be inferior to a regime of amlodipine and perindopril in the recent ASCOT study, raising further doubts about the efficacy of beta-blockers in uncomplicated hypertension.

With potential adverse effects, especially in combination with thiazide diuretics (metabolic effects, see under 'beta-blockers and diabetes'), beta-blockers are now out of favour as a first-line antihypertensive agent in uncomplicated hypertension. Indeed, beta-blockers are now removed as a first-line antihypertensive treatment in uncomplicated hypertension in the recent NICE hypertension guidelines (see later).

However, beta-blockers should not be discarded completely. They have proven symptomatic benefit in stable angina, reduce the incidence of recurrent fatal and non-fatal myocardial infarction (MI) and sudden death in patients following a first MI, and improve prognosis in patients with heart failure due to left ventricular systolic impairment (carvedilol, bisoprolol, nebivolol and extended-release metoprolol).

Therefore, beta-blockers should be used in the presence of these compelling indications, but not as first-line agent in the treatment of uncomplicated hypertension.

Adverse effects and contraindications

Most of the side-effects of beta-blockers are predictable from their pharmacology. For example, beta-blockers slow the rate of conduction at the atrioventricular node and are thus contraindicated in patients with second- and third-degree heart block. Sinus bradycardia is common and is not a reason to stop beta-blockers unless the patient is symptomatic or the heart rate falls below 40 beats/min.

Small doses of beta-blockers can cause bronchospasm due to a blockade of pulmonary beta$_2$-adrenoreceptors, although the problem is less common with cardioselective agents. Even so, all beta-blockers are contraindicated in asthma.

The blockade of beta-receptors in the peripheral circulation causes vasoconstriction at least in the immediate term, and beta-blockers therefore should be used with caution in patients with rest ischaemia of the legs. Nevertheless, they are reasonably tolerated in those with lesser degrees of peripheral vascular disease.

The lipid-soluble beta-blockers (e.g. propranolol and metoprolol) cross the blood–brain barrier more readily and are associated with a higher incidence of side-effects, including sleep disturbances and nightmares. Exercise capacity may be reduced by the beta-blockers and patients may experience tiredness and fatigue. As with most pharmacologically treated patients, impotence has been reported.

> Beta-blocker side-effects can usually be predicted, e.g. slowing the rate of conduction at the atrioventricular node, so they can be contraindicated

Beta-blockers and diabetes

Like diuretics, non-selective beta-blockers can worsen glucose intolerance and hyperlipidaemia. In diabetics prone to hypoglycaemia, beta-blockers could theoretically reduce the awareness of low blood glucose. Nevertheless, many diabetic hypertensive patients have good reasons to be on a beta-blocker, such as a previous myocardial infarction, and should not be denied them because of concerns about such metabolic side-effects.

Beta-blockers may also promote weight gain and in the CAPP study, treatment based on beta-blockers and thiazides resulted in significantly more patients (approximately 21%) developing diabetes over five years when compared to treatment based on the ACE inhibitors. However, body weight and metabolic changes did not adversely influence the efficacy of antihypertensive therapy at reducing cardiovascular morbidity and mortality. Furthermore, in the Atherosclerosis Risk in Communities Study of 12,550 adults 45–64 years old who did not have diabetes, subjects with hypertension who were taking thiazide diuretics were not at greater risk for the subsequent development of diabetes than were subjects with hypertension who were not

receiving any antihypertensive therapy (relative hazard, 0.91; 95% CI, 0.73 to 1.13). In contrast, hypertensive patients who were taking beta-blockers had a 28% higher risk of subsequent diabetes (relative hazard, 1.28; 95% CI, 1.04 to 1.57).

As discussed, the concern about the risk of diabetes should not discourage physicians from prescribing thiazide diuretics to non-diabetic adults who have hypertension. However, the concomitant use of beta-blockers does appear to increase the risk of diabetes. This potential adverse effect must therefore be weighed against the proven benefits of beta-blockers in patients with compelling indications.

Calcium antagonists

Calcium antagonists, otherwise known as calcium channel blockers, act by interfering with the action of voltage-gated calcium channels in the cell membrane, thus reducing the inflow of calcium, smooth muscle contraction and electrical conductivity.

Classes of calcium antagonist

In general, calcium antagonists may be divided into two classes. The dihydropyridines, such as nifedipine and amlodipine, act predominantly by causing peripheral vasodilatation; and the non-dihydropyridines, such as verapamil and diltiazem, which also slow the heart rate and atrioventricular node conduction. The older calcium antagonists, such as nifedipine, have short half-lives and may cause rapid vasodilatation, a reflex tachycardia and catecholamine surges, which increase adverse effects and may aggravate myocardial ischaemia. Certainly, short-acting nifedipine capsules should not be used. The tendency to crush and give them sublingually is illogical, as they are not absorbed from the buccal mucosa, and should never be used. The crushed nifedipine capsule also alters the pharmacokinetics, which can cause erratic falls in BP. Longer-acting agents such as amlodipine or slow-release preparations of nifedipine partially overcome these problems.

The phenylalkylamine calcium channel blocker verapamil is less well studied compared to dihydropyridine calcium blockers. In general, verapamil is a useful alternative to beta-blockers (for example in patients with angina) when the latter are contraindicated because of the side-effect profile or asthma. In one study, verapamil has even been shown to have synergistic effects in combination with the dihydropyridine calcium channel blocker nitrendipine.

> There are two general classes of calcium antagonists: dihydropyridines (e.g. nifedipine and amlodipine) and non-dihydropyridines (e.g. verapamil and diltiazem)

Clinical studies of calcium channel antagonists

In the mid-1990s, a series of pharmacosurveillance case-control studies suggested that the short-acting dihydropyridine calcium antagonists (such as nifedipine capsules) actually increased the risk of coronary events, cancer, bleeding, depression, suicide and other adverse events. There is little biological plausibility for some of the adverse effects proposed.

Recent data from the SYST-EUR trial demonstrated that antihypertensive treatment with the short-acting dihydropyridine calcium antagonist nitrendipine, convincingly reduced strokes and heart attacks, without an increase in conditions previously attributed to the calcium antagonists (e.g. tumours, bleeding and non-cardiac death) (Table 6.2). Recent trials (INSIGHT, NORDIL) show no significant difference between the calcium antagonists and 'conventional' antihypertensive drugs (diuretics, beta-blockers).

Pahor and colleagues (2000) published a meta-analysis of nine eligible trials that included 27,743 participants, and reported that the calcium antagonists and other drugs achieved similar control of both systolic and diastolic blood pressure. However, compared with patients assigned diuretics, beta-blockers, ACE inhibitors or clonidine ($n=15,044$), those assigned calcium antagonists ($n=12,699$) had a significantly higher risk of acute myocardial infarction (odds ratio 1.26 [95% CI 1.11–1.43], $P=0.0003$), congestive heart failure (1.25 [1.07–1.46], $P=0.005$), and major cardiovascular events (1.10 [1.02–1.18], $P=0.018$). There was no difference for the outcomes of stroke (0.90 [0.80–1.02], $P=0.10$) and all-cause mortality (1.03 [0.94–1.13], $P=0.54$).

In contrast, Staessen and colleagues (2001) published a larger meta-analysis of nine randomized trials comparing treatments in 62,605 hypertensive patients which suggested that calcium-channel blockers provided more reduction in the risk of stroke (13.5%, 95% CI 1.3–24.2, $P=0.03$) and less reduction in the risk of myocardial infarction (19.2%, 3.5–37.3,

Table 6.2
The Syst-Eur Study. (Adapted from Staessen et al. Lancet 1997; **350**: 757–64.)

	Rate/1000 patients years (number of events)		
	Placebo (n=2297)	Active (n=2398)	P value
CV events			
Stroke	10.1 (57)	5.7 (34)	0.007
Cardiac endpoints	12.6 (70)	8.5 (50)	0.03
Non-CV events			
Fatal/non-fatal cancer	14.7 (82)	12.4 (73)	0.29
Benign neoplasm	3.0 (17)	4.0 (24)	0.35

$P=0.01$). The recent ASCOT study provides further support for the use of a calcium channel blocker-based antihypertensive regime. In this study of over 19,000 patients with hypertension, amlodipine as first-line, with the addition of ACE inhibitor, was associated with lower all-cause mortality (a secondary endpoint) compared to the atenolol-based regime. Hence, the overall evidence strongly suggests that the benefits of dihydropyridine calcium antagonist treatment clearly exceed any risks.

Dihydropyridine calcium antagonists are an appropriate first-line treatment of hypertension in most cases, especially in low renin states (see later).

Adverse effects

The main side-effect with calcium antagonists is ankle oedema due to vasodilatation, which also causes headache, flushing and palpitation especially with short-acting dihydropyridines. Some side-effects can be offset by combining a calcium antagonist with a beta-blocker.

Verapamil reduces intestinal motility and can cause significant constipation, but more seriously it can cause heart block especially in those with underlying conduction problems. Verapamil should not be prescribed with a beta-blocker owing to the risk of asystole, complete heart block or heart failure. Diltiazem can similarly cause gastrointestinal and conduction problems, although less frequently than verapamil. Verapamil, diltiazem and short-acting dihydropyridines are best avoided in patients with heart failure. In contrast, the long-acting dihydropyridines, such as amlodipine and felodipine, are neutral in heart failure and would be useful for the concomitant treatment of hypertension or angina in these patients.

> The main side-effect of calcium antagonists is ankle oedema, but this can sometimes be offset by combining with a beta-blocker (though not verapamil)

Alpha$_1$-adrenoreceptor blockers

The alpha$_1$-adrenoreceptor blockers cause vasodilatation by blocking the action of noradrenaline (norepinephrine) at post-synaptic alpha$_1$-receptors in arteries and veins, resulting in a fall in peripheral resistance without a compensatory rise in cardiac output. The older alpha$_1$-blocker prazosin is short acting and tends to produce precipitate falls in BP, but the longer-acting doxazosin combines the advantage of a more gentle reduction in BP with once-daily dosing.

Alpha$_1$-adrenoreceptor blockers produce comparable reductions in BP to first-line antihypertensive drugs. They are useful as a third-line drug, producing good falls in BP where using two agents combined has failed.

In contrast to the beta-blockers and diuretics, alpha$_1$-adrenoreceptor blockers modestly improve serum, lipid and glucose tolerance, but whether or not this translates into improved outcomes is unknown, particularly with the lack of data on these agents.

> The alpha$_1$-adrenoreceptor blockers produce vasodilatation by blocking the action of noradrenaline (norepinephrine) in both arteries and veins, leading to a reduction in peripheral resistance without an equivalent compensatory increase in cardiac output

The ALLHAT trial

One worrying analysis from the ALLHAT trial on doxazosin has been highlighted. In January 2000, the independent review committee recommended termination of the doxazosin arm ($n=9067$) of ALLHAT, on account of a 25% higher rate of combined CVD, a major secondary endpoint. After four years, 86% of patients assigned to chlorthalidone were still taking the drug as opposed to 75% in the doxazosin arm, and the mean systolic BP was 135 mmHg in the chlorthalidone group and 137 mmHg in the doxazosin group. Diastolic BPs were similar in the two arms of the trial.

For doxazosin versus chlorthalidone, the relative risk (RR) of developing:

- combined CVD endpoint was 1.25 (95% CI 1.17–1.33; $P< 0.0001$)
- heart failure was 2.04 (95% CI 1.79–2.32)
- stroke was 1.19 (95% CI 1.01–1.4; $P=0.04$).

Thus, it appeared that chlorthalidone, a cheaper drug, was superior to doxazosin for hypertension control, drug compliance and reduction of cardiovascular complications.

Hence, alpha-blockers should not be used as a first-line agent.

Adverse effects

Alpha$_1$-adrenoreceptor blockers are, on the whole, well tolerated, the main side-effect being postural hypotension with the shorter-acting agents. In women, alpha$_1$-adrenoreceptor blockers may cause urinary incontinence, while in men they may improve the symptoms of benign prostatic hypertrophy. Like most antihypertensive drugs, alpha$_1$-adrenoreceptor blockers can cause headache and fatigue.

ACE inhibitors

ACE inhibitors have become increasingly popular antihypertensive agents over the past decade. They work by blocking the renin–angiotensin system, inhibiting the conversion of the inactive angiotensin I to the powerful vasoconstrictor and stimulator of aldosterone release angiotensin II. This results in decreased peripheral vascular resistance and also a reduction in the levels of the sodium-retaining hormone aldosterone.

ACE inhibitors also reduce the breakdown of the vasodilator bradykinin, which may enhance their action but is also responsible for their most troublesome side-effect of coughing. Furthermore, ACE inhibitors may improve endothelial function and reduce central adrenergic tone. They also have beneficial effects on renal haemodynamics, reducing

intraglomerular hypertension and causing improvements in proteinuric renal disease.

> ACE inhibitors work by blocking the renin–angiotensin system, inhibiting the conversion of angiotensin I to angiotensin II

ACE inhibitors and the renin–angiotensin system

Because ACE inhibitors are competitive inhibitors of ACE, the secondary increase in levels of angiotensin I (due to loss of negative feedback) can overcome the ACE blockade. This leads to the return of angiotensin II levels to normal. It is also probable that other non-ACE pathways (involving chymases and tissue plasminogen activator) facilitate the conversion of angiotensin I to angiotensin II and consequent elevation of aldosterone levels. This is termed 'ACE escape' and accounts for the failure of ACE inhibitors to comprehensively block the renin–angiotensin system.

ACE inhibitors as single agents in treatment of hypertension

ACE inhibitors are effective as single agents in hypertension. There is generally little to choose between the large number of ACE inhibitors available. The Captopril Prevention Project (CAPP) study demonstrated that captopril was as effective as traditional antihypertensive agents (mainly thiazides and beta-blockers) in preventing adverse outcomes in hypertension. Other ACE inhibitors, such as fosinopril and trandolapril, have the advantage of hepatic as well as renal excretion. Perindopril, lisinopril and trandolapril are agents with long half-lives, and provide good 24-hour antihypertensive coverage.

Clinical studies of ACE inhibitors

The prognostic benefit of ACE inhibitors is well established in patients with heart failure due to left ventricular systolic dysfunction (CONSENSUS, SAVE and SOLVD trials). Similarly, patients with heart failure post-MI derive significant benefit from ACE inhibition (ramipril in AIRE and trandolapril in TRACE). The positive findings from these early trials led to studies of ACE inhibition in patients at high cardiovascular risk without heart failure.

The HOPE trial randomized 9297 patients at high cardiovascular risk to ramipril or placebo and demonstrated significant reductions in death, MI and stroke. The EUROPA study randomized over 12,000 patients to perindopril or placebo and demonstrated significant reductions in the composite endpoint of cardiovascular death and non-fatal MI. However, there was no significant difference between trandolapril and placebo in cardiovascular death and non-fatal MI in the PEACE trial of 8290 patients. The negative findings in the PEACE trial probably reflect the lower risk profile of the patients in that study (higher use of lipid-lowering treatment and coronary revascularization). Indeed, cardiovascular death and non-fatal MI were highest in the placebo arm of the HOPE study cohort (8.1% and 12.3%), followed by the placebo arm of the EUROPA cohort (4.1% and 6.2%) and lowest in the PEACE cohort (3.7% and 5.3%). Hence, the benefit of ACE inhibitors may be related to the level of cardiovascular risk, with particular benefit in patients with established cardiovascular disease at high risk of further cardiovascular events.

ACE inhibitors are also used in patients with left ventricular dysfunction, and this class is likely to be the most efficacious in LVH regression. The ECG-LVH substudy from the HOPE trial compared baseline and end-of-study ECGs from 8281 patients at high cardiovascular risk who were randomized to ramipril or placebo and followed for 4.5 years in the main HOPE trial. In this analysis, ramipril prevented LVH, or caused a gradual regression of LVH, in 91.9% of patients; interestingly, however, 90.2% of patients assigned to placebo also had regression or prevention of LVH. Patients who experienced regression or prevention of LVH had a reduced risk of the predefined primary outcome

(cardiovascular death, MI, stroke) and of congestive heart failure. Importantly, this effect was independent of hypertension or blood pressure reduction.

ACE inhibitors are also useful in diabetic hypertensive patients, where they slow the progression of diabetic nephropathy (ramipril reduced progression of albuminuria in micro-HOPE study). Reduction in the progression of nephropathy in patients with type 1 diabetes has also been demonstrated (Lewis et al. and EUCLID). Furthermore, these agents have shown some benefits in improving diabetic retinopathy and possibly even diabetic neuropathy.

The combination of ACE inhibitor and diuretic has also been shown to reduce the risk of stroke. The PROGRESS study included 6105 patients with a previous history of stroke or transient ischaemic attack and demonstrated significant 43% reduction in the risk of stroke in patients treated with a combination of perindopril and indapamide. The benefit of this combination treatment was associated with significant reduction in blood pressure of 12/5 mmHg. Interestingly, a subgroup analysis of this study found no significant reduction in the risk of stroke with perindopril alone.

Based on these studies, ACE inhibitors are indicated in patients with heart failure from left ventricular systolic dysfunction (including post-MI), high-risk patients with CVD (especially if BP is not adequately controlled to a target of 130/80 mmHg) and patients with diabetes complicated by nephropathy. ACE inhibitors, in combination with a thiazide diuretic, are also indicated in patients with a history of stroke/TIA (secondary prevention). In addition, a number of studies suggest that ACE inhibitors may have additional benefit in reducing the incidence of new-onset diabetes, and may be recommended in patients at high risk of developing diabetes (e.g. glucose intolerance, metabolic syndrome and strong family history of diabetes).

ACE inhibitors may be most useful for treating patients with heart failure or left ventricular hypertrophy, as well as diabetic hypertensive patients

However, the ACE inhibitors tend to be less effective as antihypertensive agents in Afro-Caribbean patients and the elderly, owing to the low renin state of these patients. This relative ineffectiveness can be overcome by using high doses or adding a diuretic. The African American Study of Kidney Disease and Hypertension (AASK) trial had to be terminated early because the ACE inhibitor ramipril resulted in a significant delay in end-stage renal disease when compared with the calcium antagonist amlodipine. Patients with a relatively low renin state should not be deprived of ACE inhibitor therapy in the presence of a compelling indication.

Hence, ACE inhibitors may be used as first-line therapy in patients with higher renin state (younger and non-Afro-Caribbean patients) or in the presence of compelling indications described above.

Adverse effects

Although ACE inhibitors are successful drugs, they do have some disadvantages. ACE is not a specific enzyme and is involved in the breakdown of many other substances, such as bradykinin. The use of ACE inhibitors results in increased levels of bradykinin, resulting in the common side-effect of coughs and the less common (but serious) complication of angioedema. Coughing is more common in women and older patients. Angioedema occurs in 0.1–0.2% of patients.

Serum urea and creatinine should be checked before and a few weeks after starting an ACE inhibitor. As previously described, a rise in serum creatinine is common with the use of ACE inhibitors. In general, a rise in serum creatinine

of up to 30% that stabilizes within the first two months of treatment is acceptable and may in fact be associated with long-term preservation of renal function. However, dramatic and continued deterioration in renal function can occur in patients with bilateral renal artery stenosis. Repeated monitoring of renal function is therefore important to avoid inappropriate use or withdrawal of ACE inhibitor therapy.

Significant first-dose hypotension is a fairly uncommon side-effect of ACE inhibitors, although large doses of short-acting captopril can cause sudden falls in BP. This first-dose effect is most common in those with volume depletion such as heart failure or in patients on large doses of diuretics. The limited data available suggest that perindopril is least likely to cause this initial hypotension.

Because of their effect of reducing aldosterone and thus potassium excretion, the ACE inhibitors can also cause hyperkalaemia. Rarer side-effects of the ACE inhibitors include rash, taste disturbance, blood dyscrasias and vasculitis.

Using ACE inhibitors can lead to increased levels of bradykinin, which has the side-effect of coughs and the complication of angioedema

Angiotensin II antagonists

Antagonism of the renin–angiotensin system has become an attractive target for pharmacological intervention in light of the impressive record of ACE inhibitors, most notably with angiotensin II antagonists. Angiotensin II, an octapeptide derived from its inactive precursor angiotensin I by the action of ACE, is the final product of the renin–angiotensin system. Angiotensin II antagonists block the action of angiotensin II at its peripheral receptors, which offers the prospect of overcoming the 'ACE escape' phenomenon (see under ACE inhibitors and the renin–angiotensin system).

Mode of action

Angiotensin II is a significant contributor to the pathogenesis of arterial disease, hypertension, LVH, heart failure and renal disease. Whereas ACE inhibitors work by reducing the conversion of angiotensin I to angiotensin II, the angiotensin II antagonists block the action of angiotensin II at its peripheral receptors, particularly the type I angiotensin II (ATI) receptor. This results in elevated angiotensin II levels via a loss of feedback, which may lead to increased activation of the type II angiotensin II (ATII) receptors as ATI receptors are blocked. Reduced activation of ATI and increased activation of ATII receptors are believed to be the key mechanism of benefit of angiotensin II antagonist therapy. Angiotensin II antagonists also differ from ACE inhibitors in that they do not inhibit bradykinin breakdown, which spares them the ACE inhibitor-related cough but may lack the additional physiological benefits of bradykinin (a vasodilator). Hence, although both ACE inhibitors and angiotensin II antagonists inhibit the renin–angiotensin system, their different mechanisms of action may lead to different physiological effects, which may be of clinical relevance.

Angiotensin II antagonists lower BP by decreasing peripheral vascular resistance without affecting heart rate and cardiac output. Overall, angiotensin II antagonists produce similar falls in BP compared to ACE inhibitors. As with the ACE inhibitors, they are somewhat less effective in patients with low levels of renin, such as Afro-Carribeans and the elderly, but their action may be potentiated by the addition of a diuretic.

Clinical studies of angiotensin II antagonists

The LIFE study, reported in 2002, randomized 9193 patients with hypertension and documented LVH to losartan and atenolol, and followed up for a mean of 4.8 years. This study of high-risk hypertensive patients showed a significantly lower incidence of fatal and non-

fatal cardiovascular events in the losartan group, dominated by significant reduction in the incidence of fatal and non-fatal strokes. This study clearly demonstrates the superiority of losartan over atenolol in hypertension (see 'Efficacy of beta-blockers').

The SCOPE study randomized 4964 (older) patients with hypertension (mean age of 76 years) to candesartan or placebo. As this study permitted open-label treatment, antihypertensive treatment was used extensively in the placebo group. Unlike the LIFE study, the incidence of fatal and non-fatal CVD was not statistically significant between the two groups, though the incidence of stroke tended to be lower in the candesartan group ($P=0.06$).

The VALUE trial is the largest trial of angiotensin II antagonists in hypertension to date. This study randomized 15,245 patients to valsartan or amlodipine and followed up over 4.2 years. The primary endpoint of cardiac morbidity and mortality was not significantly different, although more myocardial infarctions ($P=0.02$) and strokes ($P=0.08$) were observed in the valsartan group. The consistently higher BP in the valsartan group may have accounted for these findings. Overall, these studies suggest that angiotensin II antagonists are likely to be as effective as other classes of antihypertensive therapy (probably with the exception of atenolol) and the degree of BP lowering is the key determinant of cardiovascular outcomes.

Angiotensin II antagonists have also been studied in patients with chronic heart failure, post-MI heart failure and diabetic nephropathy. In chronic heart failure, angiotensin II antagonists have not been shown to be superior to ACE inhibitors (valsartan in Val-HeFT, losartan in ELITE II) although candesartan may offer cardiovascular benefits in patients intolerant of ACE inhibitors (CHARM-alternative). Similarly, angiotensin II antagonists have not been shown to be superior to ACE inhibitors in post-MI heart failure (valsartan was not inferior to captopril in

VALIANT, but cardiovascular mortality was higher in losartan compared with captopril in OPTIMAAL). Angiotensin II antagonists have been shown to reduce the progression of (type 2) diabetic nephropathy (losartan in RENAAL, valsartan in MARVAL, irbesartan in IDNT and IRMA-2).

Based on these data, angiotensin II antagonists cannot be recommended over ACE inhibitors in patients with heart failure. However, the data support the use of angiotensin II antagonists in patients with heart failure (after MI), who are ACE inhibitor-intolerant, patients with type 2 diabetes complicated by nephropathy and patients with hypertension with LVH. Indeed, these represent compelling indications for angiotensin II antagonists in the 2004 British Hypertension Society guidelines. Like ACE inhibitors, angiotensin II antagonists appear to reduce the incidence of type 2 diabetes.

Like ACE inhibitors, angiotensin II antagonists may be used as first-line therapy in patients with higher renin state (younger and non-Afro-Caribbean patients) or in the presence of compelling indications described above.

Adverse effects

The main advantage of the angiotensin II antagonists is their apparent lack of side-effects. One study compared losartan with ACE inhibitors, beta-blockers and calcium channel blockers. The results indicated that using losartan, the incidence of any drug-related adverse experience (including cough) was similar to that of placebo. First-dose hypotension occurred in only 0.4% with losartan 50 mg.

Very rarely, however, angioedema has been reported with losartan. Like the ACE inhibitors, the angiotensin II antagonists may cause hyperkalaemia, renal impairment and hypotension, and are contraindicated in patients with renal artery stenosis. Otherwise they are almost as well tolerated as placebo.

> Angiotensin II antagonists are well tolerated and infrequently cause any significant side-effects

Other antihypertensive agents

Other (older) antihypertensive drugs still have a role in some special situations (e.g. pregnancy) and in resistant hypertension. Because they are cheap, they are popular in countries where hypertensive patients on low incomes have to pay for their own medication. *They are not recommended as first-line treatment of uncomplicated hypertension.*

Centrally acting antihypertensive drugs

Centrally acting agents, such as clonidine and methyldopa, have previously been used to treat hypertension. These agents reduce sympathetic outflow by stimulating alpha$_2$-adrenoreceptors in the central nervous system. This effect leads to a fall in both cardiac output and peripheral vascular resistance. Indeed, methyldopa is safe in the hypertensive pregnant woman, and is commonly used in such patients.

Moxonidine represents the first of a new class of centrally acting antihypertensive drugs, the selective imidazoline receptor agonists, and is hoped to have the beneficial effects of centrally acting drugs without their side-effects. By stimulating central imidazoline receptors, moxonidine also reduces central sympathetic outflow, without the dry mouth and sedation of central alpha$_2$-receptor blockade. Moxonidine also reduces peripheral vascular resistance without an increase in heart rate. The drug may also decrease plasma renin activity by direct action on the kidney, and might increase the excretion of sodium and water. Moxonidine has been shown to be superior to placebo and comparable to the main classes of antihypertensive drugs in lowering BP. There are no long-term studies with survival or cardiovascular events as endpoints, and one trial in heart failure (MOXCON) showed an increase in adverse effects compared to placebo, and was stopped early.

Mode of action and side-effects

Side-effects include sedation, a dry mouth and fluid retention. The older agents also suffer from the problem of rebound hypertension on withdrawal. Furthermore, methyldopa can also cause autoimmune hepatic derangement and haemolytic anaemia. Moxonidine causes fewer problems with dry mouth than clonidine, but other side-effects such as sedation, headache, nausea and sleep disturbance may occur. Overall, moxonidine appears to be as well tolerated as the main classes of antihypertensive drugs. Moxonidine also has no adverse effects on plasma lipids and glucose.

> Moxonidine stimulates the central imidazoline receptors and reduces central sympathetic outflow, without the dry mouth and sedation side-effects of central alpha$_2$-receptor blockade. However, headache, nausea and interrupted sleep may occur

In summary, moxonidine is an effective antihypertensive agent, but although an improvement over clonidine it has not been demonstrated to have major advantages over more well-established drugs.

Direct vasodilators

The direct vasodilators (e.g. hydralazine, minoxidil) act directly to relax vascular smooth muscle, thereby reducing peripheral vascular resistance. The resulting activation of the sympathetic nervous system means that their use is commonly associated with reflex tachycardia and can only successfully be used in combination with drugs that block sympathetic activity. The combination of hydralazine and nitrates has proven of benefit in heart failure due to systolic dysfunction and may be better than ACE inhibitors for hypertensive Afro-Caribbean patients who develop heart failure. Hydralazine use may be complicated by the development of systemic lupus erythematosus, while hypertrichosis may be troublesome with minoxidil (not suitable for women). All these drugs may cause rapid falls in blood pressure.

Adrenergic neuron blockers

Such agents are now rarely used in the UK. Reserpine and guanethidine inhibit the release of noradrenaline (norepinephrine) from peripheral nerves, thus reducing sympathetic tone, peripheral vascular resistance and cardiac output. They cause postural hypotension and central nervous system depression. Where low costs are paramount, especially in the Third World, small doses of reserpine combined with a diuretic form an effective regimen.

Multifactorial interventions to prevent cardiovascular disease

Blood pressure should be managed in the context of overall risk. The importance of considering serum cholesterol, although obvious, has been much neglected. Indeed, hypertensive patients tend to have higher cholesterol levels than the general population and it is well recognized that those with both raised BP and raised cholesterol are at particularly high risk of cardiovascular events. As long ago as 1987, it was found that treating hypertension alone in patients with raised cholesterol had little impact on cardiovascular events.

The treatment of hypercholesterolaemia has been transformed by the introduction of the 3-hydroxy-3-methylgluteryl coenzyme A reductase inhibitors (statins). The value of statins in secondary and primary prevention in high-risk patients has previously been demonstrated. The more recent lipid-lowering arm of the ASCOT study was terminated early due to significant reductions in cardiovascular events with atorvastatin in hypertensive patients with even modestly raised cholesterol levels. This confirms the value of addressing multiple risk factors in the treatment of all patients with hypertension.

The anti-platelet agent aspirin has long been used in the treatment and secondary prevention of many of the complications of hypertension, but until recently, little information has been available on its role in the management of the asymptomatic hypertensive individual. Warfarin has also been found to be useful as a thromboprophylaxis in hypertensive patients with atrial fibrillation, but if BPs remain uncontrolled, such therapy carries significant risks, especially from intracranial haemorrhage.

> The importance of combined interventions has been recognized for some time, although the importance of taking serum cholesterol into account had been ignored

Aspirin

Despite the strong pathophysiological and epidemiological associations between thrombosis and hypertension, there were few or no data on the routine use of antithrombotic therapy in hypertension until the recent publication of the Hypertension Optimal Treatment (HOT) trial.

There are good reasons for treating hypertensive patients with antithrombotic therapy, especially when there have been previous heart attacks and strokes, i.e. secondary prevention. Examples include the use of aspirin following myocardial infarction and cerebral infarction, and warfarin if concomitant atrial fibrillation is present.

HOT trial

There are no trials on the use of warfarin as primary prevention in uncomplicated hypertensive patients as such. The HOT trial was the first study to investigate the use of aspirin as primary prevention in hypertension.

In the HOT trial, 75 mg of aspirin was given daily to treated hypertensive patients aged 50 years or above. This reduced cardiovascular events by 15% and myocardial infarction by 36%, but had no effect on fatal events. This study showed the potential of aspirin to prevent 1.5 myocardial infarctions per 1000 hypertensive patients per year, which was in addition to the benefit achieved by lowering the BP.

The benefit seen in terms of reduced cardiovascular events was at the price of a higher incidence of bleeding events in the aspirin group. There was no increase in the number of fatal bleeding events (seven events in patients taking aspirin, compared to eight in the placebo group). However, there was a 1.8% increase of non-fatal major bleeding events (129 events in patients taking aspirin, compared to 70 in the placebo group) and minor bleeds (156 and 87 respectively). These were mostly gastrointestinal and nasal. This increase in bleeding events was similar to that seen in other studies of aspirin (Figure 6.2).

> Aspirin can prevent up to 1.5 myocardial infarctions per 1000 hypertensive patients each year

Thrombosis prevention trial

In the thrombosis prevention trial of aspirin 75 mg daily for primary prevention, 26% of those studied had treated hypertension. The outcome was similar to that of the HOT trial; a 16% reduction in all cardiovascular events, 20%

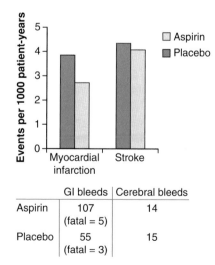

	GI bleeds	Cerebral bleeds
Aspirin	107 (fatal = 5)	14
Placebo	55 (fatal = 3)	15

Figure 6.2
Results from the HOT trial investigating the use of aspirin as primary prevention in hypertension. GI, gastrointestinal.

reduction in myocardial infarction and no effect on fatal events. In both trials, the number of clinically significant bleeding episodes caused by aspirin was similar to the number of cardiovascular events prevented by aspirin, suggesting that the margin between benefit and harm was narrow.

It should also be noted that the HOT trial studied well-controlled hypertensive patients, and in the thrombosis prevention trial, aspirin was withheld when BP was above 170/100 mmHg. Furthermore, those who developed cerebral haemorrhage in the thrombosis prevention trial had significantly higher systolic BP before the adverse event (158 mmHg, versus 135 mmHg in those with no stroke).

Thus, hypertension must be well controlled (BP <150/90 mmHg) before starting aspirin treatment for the primary prevention of CVD.

The British Hypertension Society guidelines state that 'aspirin 75 mg daily' is recommended for hypertensive patients who have:

- no contraindication to aspirin
- secondary prevention of cardiovascular complications:
  —myocardial infarction
  —angina
  —non-haemorrhagic cerebrovascular disease
  —peripheral vascular disease
  —atherosclerotic renovascular disease
- primary prevention:
  —BP controlled to <150/90 mmHg (audit standard)
  —age ≥ 50 years and target organ damage (e.g. LVH, renal impairment or proteinuria)
  —an estimated 10-year CVD risk ≥ 20% by Joint British Societies risk chart.

This includes patients with type-2 diabetes.

(Source: British Hypertension Society, 2004)

The 2004 British Hypertension Society guidelines make the point that patients with an estimated 10-year CVD risk of ≥ 20% will have their cardiovascular risk reduced by 25% using antihypertensive treatment. The addition of aspirin further reduces the risk of major cardiovascular events by 15%, giving a NNT for five years of about 90 for one cardiovascular complication and 60 for one myocardial infarction prevented by aspirin.

HMG CoA reductase inhibitors (statins)

Several primary and secondary prevention outcome trials have shown that statin treatment for primary and secondary prevention reduces major coronary events by 30%, reduces all-cause mortality significantly, and is safe, simple and well tolerated. Importantly, statin treatment substantially reduces the risk of stroke in patients who have CHD, which is an effect not seen in previous trials of lipid-lowering with non-statin drugs.

Thus, statin treatment should be targeted at a specified threshold of cardiovascular risk and *not just* at thresholds of lipid values. None the less, monitoring of lipid levels is relevant as the benefit of statin therapy is proportional to the reduction in cholesterol, especially LDL cholesterol. The current British Hypertension Society and Joint British Societies guidelines recommend statin treatment for estimated CVD risk of at least 20% and most patients with diabetes. Total cholesterol of <4 mmol/L or LDL cholesterol of <2 mmol/L are the recommended targets.

Resistant hypertension

In view of new BP targets and the need for many drugs to achieve these lower BPs, many patients will be labelled by clinicians as having 'resistant' or 'refractory' hypertension, although careful examination would reveal that such a simplistic approach may be fraught with problems.

A large data review from the USA (the National Health and Nutrition Examination Survey) has demonstrated that only 55% of hypertensive patients are being treated and only 29% have reached a target BP of 140/90 mmHg. Failure to achieve these goals can be attributed to several underlying causes, one of them being refractory hypertension. However, any debate about resistant hypertension is hampered by the lack of a generally approved definition.

One definition for 'resistant' hypertension is when a rational triple combination of antihypertensive drugs in appropriate doses fails to achieve adequate BP control (BP <140/90 mmHg).

The extent of this problem becomes clear when considering that up to 85% of patients referred to specialist hypertension clinics are reported to have 'resistant' hypertension when similar criteria to those above are used.

> Diagnosing resistant hypertension is made more difficult by the lack of a standard definition

Factors contributing to resistance

Several factors contribute to treatment resistance (Table 6.3). In primary care, truly resistant hypertension is most commonly caused by drug non-compliance. This is not an inconsequential problem as non-compliance rates of up to 50% have been reported with antihypertensive therapy. This is particularly a problem in younger patients who do not fully appreciate the need to treat what is usually an asymptomatic disease or risk factor. However, drug side-effects and multiple drug dosing need to be carefully excluded as possible reasons for non-compliance – simple measures such as a change in drug class and the use of once-daily dosing may help. Patient education and greater awareness of the risks associated with hypertension are also needed.

Other causes of resistant hypertension

Other causes of resistant hypertension include concomitant medication, secondary

Table 6.3
Causes of lack of response to therapy

- Non-adherence to therapy:
  —instructions not clear and/or not given to patient in writing
  —inadequate or no patient education
  —lack of involvement of patient in treatment plan
  —cost of medication
  —side-effects of medication
  —organic brain syndrome (e.g. memory deficit)
  —inconvenient dosing
- Drug-related causes:
  —dosage too low
  —inappropriate combinations (e.g. two centrally acting adrenergic inhibitors)
  —rapid inactivation (e.g. hydralazine)
  —drug interactions
  —non-steroidal anti-inflammatory drugs
  —oral contraceptives
  —sympathomimetics
  —antidepressants
  —adrenal steroids
  —nasal decongestants
  —liquorice-containing substances (e.g. chewing tobacco)
  —cocaine or other illicit drugs
  —cyclosporine
  —erythropoietin
- Associated conditions:
  —increasing obesity
  —alcohol intake >1 ounce/day of ethanol
- Secondary hypertension:
  —renal insufficiency
  —renovascular hypertension
  —phaeochromocytoma
  —primary aldosteronism
- Volume overload:
  —inadequate diuretic therapy
  —excessive sodium intake
  —fluid retention from reduction of blood pressure
  —progressive renal damage
- Pseudohypertension
- 'White-coat' effect

(Adapted from Seventh report of the Joint National Committee on Detection, Evaluation, and Treatment of High Blood Pressure (JNC VII). *Hypertension* 2003; **42**: 1206–52.)

hypertension, obesity, alcohol misuse and white-coat hypertension, which may be excluded by thorough clinical assessment and simple laboratory investigations. An approach to resistant hypertension is summarized in Table 6.4.

Overall, the prevalence of secondary causes of hypertension amounts to about 5%, but investigations for rare underlying causes should be reserved for those patients whose initial assessment results are indicative of a secondary cause, or in patients with an unusual clinical presentation (e.g. before the age of 20 years, after the age of 50 years, marked end-organ damage, BP >180/110 mmHg). The patient's BP response to treatment can sometimes point to secondary causes. Sudden development of renal failure or dramatic reduction in BP following treatment with an ACE inhibitor or angiotensin II receptor blocker would be consistent with renal artery stenosis.

White-coat hypertension

White-coat hypertension should be suspected in patients with resistant hypertension but no evidence of target organ damage. Some studies have suggested that up to 50% of patients referred to specialized clinics for assessment of their resistant hypertension had normotensive ambulatory BP readings. In hypertensive patients, there can also be a significant difference between office and ambulatory BP, the so-called 'white-coat effect'. If present, the readings in a clinical setting can exceed ambulatory readings by at least 20/10 mmHg.

Obesity, alcohol intake and cigarette smoking

A variety of other patient-related factors can contribute to resistant hypertension. Obesity is a 'pro-hypertensive' condition and weight loss of 10.4 kg reduces the mean arterial BP by 10/8 mmHg. There also seems to be a J-shaped relationship between alcohol and hypertension, where every unit of alcohol in excess of two units a day increases the BP by approximately 1 mmHg. Conversely, a reduction of alcohol intake in regular drinkers lowers BP by 4 mmHg. Another risk factor for resistant hypertension is cigarette smoking, which causes a pressor response and thereby increases the BP.

Pseudohypertension

'Pseudohypertension' might be another underlying cause of resistant hypertension. In pseudohypertension, cuff sphygmomanometer BP readings are falsely elevated when compared to (normal) intra-arterial pressures. This condition is a manifestation of sclerosis of the brachial artery and is more common in the elderly. It should be suspected if the Osler's manoeuvre is positive, i.e. when a palpable radial pulse is present when the cuff is inflated above the systolic BP. However, the only reliable way of proving pseudohypertension is measurement of intra-arterial BP.

Concomitant medication

Concomitant medication is a frequently neglected cause of treatment-resistant hypertension. For example, chronic non-steroidal anti-inflammatory drug (NSAID) use increases the risk of developing hypertension and can impair the success rate of antihypertensive medication. NSAIDs can increase mean BP by about 4–5 mmHg. In addition to this hypertensive property, NSAIDs antagonize the effects of most antihypertensive drug classes. These effects are particularly important as NSAIDs are widely available without needing to be prescribed. Only careful history taking with direct questioning about NSAIDs can reveal this problem.

Response to drug therapy – the renin state

A further important cause of resistant hypertension is a suboptimal antihypertensive treatment regimen. The choice of the first-line drug is very much influenced by the patient's age, ethnicity and coexisting disease(s), and initiation should follow or coincide with non-pharmacological methods, such as dietary advice, exercise and weight loss.

A variable response to the four major antihypertensive drug classes has been noted. In particular, age and ethnic influences on the renin–angiotensin system are of relevance. For example, patients aged <50 years are more likely to respond to ACE inhibitors and beta-blockers, whereas calcium channel blockers and thiazide diuretics are more effective in patients aged >50 years. These age-related differences can be explained by a different activation status of the renin–angiotensin system, with plasma renin activity declining with age.

Thus, blockade of the renin–angiotensin system with the ACE inhibitors, angiotensin II receptor antagonists or beta-blockers tends to be more effective in young patients, who are more likely to have higher renin activity. In contrast, the diuretics and calcium channel blockers are first-line agents in patients with low renin states, such as the elderly and Afro-Caribbeans. This forms the basis for the 'Birmingham Square' and the current British Hypertension Society ABCD algorithm.

> Age and ethnic origin can influence the patient's response to drug therapy

Combination antihypertensive therapy

Many patients will not have their BP controlled by one drug alone. As most antihypertensive agents have fairly flat dose–response curves, using large doses of a single agent will produce significant increases in side-effects without much further lowering of BP. The solution to these problems is to use a combination of two or more drugs. Indeed, the American JNC-VII guidelines suggest that 'when BP is more than 20 mmHg above systolic goal or 10 mmHg above diastolic goal, consideration should be given to initiate therapy with 2 drugs'. In general, about half of hypertensive patients will require two drugs and one-third may require three or more drugs.

In the HOT study, for example, fewer than one-third of hypertensive patients were controlled by monotherapy and more than one-third required a combination of three or more drugs to achieve optimal BP control. The major classes of drug generally have additive effects on BP when they are prescribed together, and most hypertensive people will require combinations of antihypertensive therapy to achieve optimal BP control.

> Combination of submaximal doses of two drugs results in larger BP responses and fewer side-effects than maximal doses of a single drug

Drug combinations

Effective combination therapy will use drugs with different (and complementary) primary modes of action. In general, the combination should include one effective against a high renin state and another for a low renin state. Such combinations include:

- a diuretic with an ACE inhibitor (or angiotensin II antagonist)
- a calcium antagonist with an ACE inhibitor (or angiotensin II antagonist)

As previously discussed, beta-blockers are not recommended for the initial treatment of hypertension in the absence of compelling indications (see under 'Beta-adrenergic receptor blockers').

For third-line drug therapy, commonly used combinations are diuretic, ACE inhibitor and calcium antagonist. Additional antihypertensive therapy beyond these three agents is less established. Alpha-receptor blockers or centrally acting agents such as moxonidine or methyldopa can be considered, but there are few data confirming their effectiveness and possible side-effects in combination therapy. Spironolactone is also increasingly used as 'add-on' therapy, although careful monitoring of renal function and serum potassium is mandatory. Specialist referral should be considered in these patients with 'resistant hypertension'.

Fixed-dose combinations are not widely used in the UK. These combinations are convenient for patients and acceptable provided they are used as second-line treatment when monotherapy is ineffective, the individual drug components are appropriate and there are no major cost implications.

Concomitant disease states should also influence sensible prescribing (Table 6.5). For example, patients with diabetes mellitus should receive ACE inhibitors because of the particularly favourable effects on nephropathy, retinopathy and LVH. Based upon the strength of evidence for reduction of cardiovascular mortality, a sensible choice as first-line drug therapy seems to be:

- ACE inhibitor/angiotensin II antagonist in the young
- a thiazide diuretic (or calcium channel blocker) in elderly or Afro-Caribbean patients

Table 6.5
Useful antihypertensive agents in patients with concomitant conditions

Condition	Possible agents
Benign prostatic hypertrophy	Alpha-blockers
Hyperthyroidism	Beta-blockers
Migraine	Beta-blockers
Atrial fibrillation	Beta-blockers, verapamil, diltiazem
Osteoporosis	Diuretics

- ACE inhibitor in the presence of concomitant heart failure
- beta-blockers or ACE inhibitors in patients with coronary artery disease
- ACE inhibitors in people with diabetes.

> The most effective combination therapy uses drugs with different primary modes of action, so that the side-effects of one drug may be overcome by the action of another

Clinical guidelines

The British Hypertension Society (BHS) amended the 1999 guidelines and published new recommendations in 2004 based on new clinical data. The publication of the ASCOT study in 2005 prompted the National Institute of Clinical Excellence (NICE) to update the recommendations for antihypertensive therapy. Therefore, the 2004 BHS antihypertensive treatment algorithm (ABCD) (see Figure 6.4) is now superseded by the 2006 NICE algorithm (see Figure 6.5). The 2004 BHS treatment algorithm is provided below for reference.

A summary of the 2004 British Hypertension Society guidelines
Threshold for antihypertensive therapy

- Use non-pharmacological measures in all patients with hypertension and people with borderline hypertension.
- Initiate antihypertensive drug therapy in people with sustained systolic BP ≥ 160 mmHg or sustained diastolic BP ≥ 100 mmHg (Figure 6.3).
- Decide on treatment in people with sustained systolic BP between 140 and 159 mmHg or sustained diastolic BP between 90 and 99 mmHg according to the presence or absence of target organ damage, diabetes, established CVD or an estimated 10-year CVD risk of ≥ 20% (according to the Joint British Societies risk assessment chart).

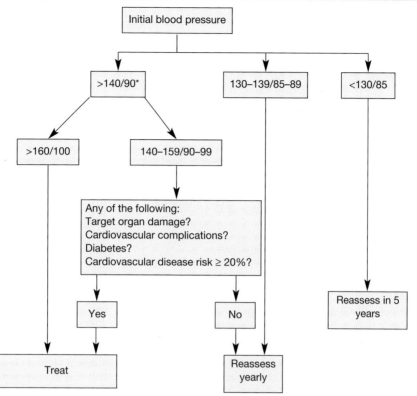

*If initial BP >180/110, confirm over 1–2 weeks unless malignant phase hypertension
If initial BP 160–179/100–109, confirm over 3–4 weeks then treat
If initial BP 140–159/90–99, confirm over 12 weeks then treat

Figure 6.3
Blood pressure threshold for intervention. (Adapted from Williams B, Poulter NR, Brown MJ, et al. Guidelines for management of hypertension: report of the fourth working party of the British Hypertension Society. *J Hum Hypertens* 2004; **18**: 139–85.)

Blood pressure treatment targets

- In patients with hypertension but without diabetes, optimal BP treatment targets are systolic BP <140 mmHg and diastolic BP <85 mmHg.
- In patients with hypertension and diabetes, renal disease or established cardiovascular disease, optimal BP targets are systolic BP <130 mmHg and diastolic BP <80 mmHg.

Antihypertensive treatment algorithm

- In the absence of contraindications or compelling indications (Table 6.6) for other antihypertensive agents, first-line therapy for hypertension should follow the ABCD algorithm** (Figure 6.4).
- For most patients, a combination of antihypertensive drugs will be required to achieve the recommended targets for BP

Table 6.6
Compelling indications and contraindications of antihypertensive agents

Class of drugs	Compelling indications	Contraindications
Alpha-blockers	BPH	Urinary incontinence
ACE inhibitors	Heart failure, LV dysfunction or established coronary heart disease, type-1 diabetic nephropathy, secondary stroke prevention (with thiazide)	Pregnancy, renovascular disease
Angiotensin II antagonist	ACE inhibitor intolerance (heart failure), type 2 diabetic nephropathy, hypertension with LVH	Pregnancy, renovascular disease
Beta-blockers	Myocardial infarction, angina, heart failure	Asthma or COPD, heart block
Dihydropyridine calcium channel blocker	Elderly patients, isolated systolic hypertension angina	–
Rate-limiting (non-dihydropyridine) calcium channel blocker	Angina	Heart block, heart failure
Thiazide diretics	Elderly patients, isolated systolic hypertension, heart failure, secondary stroke prevention	Gout

- ACE inhibitors and angiotensin II antagonists should be used with caution in patients with renal impairment; ACE inhibitors and angiotensin II antagonists may be preferred in patients at high risk of developing diabetes (e.g. glucose intolerance, metabolic syndrome and family history of diabetes)
- the use of beta-blockers in heart failure may lead to transient deterioration in symptoms
- thiazides may precipitate gout and concomitant allopurinol should be considered

control. The combination of beta-blocker and thiazide diuretics should be used with caution, especially in patients at high risk of developing diabetes (e.g. family history of diabetes, obesity, patients with glucose intolerance and patients of South Asian and Afro-Caribbean descent).

- Low-dose aspirin (75 mg/day) is recommended for secondary prevention or primary prevention in patients at high CVD risk (estimated CVD risk over 20%) in whom BP is controlled to the audit standard (150/90 mmHg).
- Statins are recommended for all patients with hypertension complicated by cardiovascular disease or patients at high CVD risk (estimated CVD risk over 20%).

(Adapted from William *et al. J Human Hypertens* 2004; **18**: 139–85.)

**Beta-blockers are now not recommended as first-line antihypertensive therapy for uncomplicated essential hypertension. The ACD algorithm should replace the ABCD algorithm by the BHS (see 'NICE guidelines update 2006').*

NICE guidelines update 2006

A number of studies comparing different classes of antihypertensive therapy have now been reported since the publication of the last British Hypertension Society guidelines in 2004. In 2006 the National Institute of Clinical Excellence (NICE) produced a partial update of the initial NICE guidelines published in 2004 to take these studies into consideration.

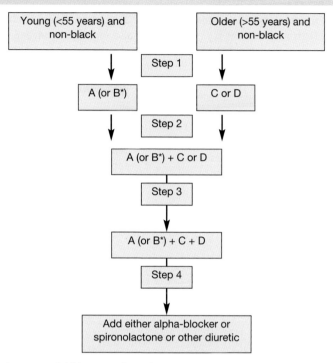

A: angiotensin-converting enzyme inhibitor or angiotensin II antagonist, B: beta-blockers, C: calcium channel blockers, D: diuretic (thiazide)
*combination of B and D may induce more new-onset diabetes compared to other combination therapy
†See Figure 6.5 for the updated treatment algorithm for hypertension (NICE update, 2006)

Figure 6.4
The ABCD algorithm for hypertension (BHS guidelines, 2004).† (Adapted from Williams B, Poulter NR, Brown MJ, et al. Guidelines for management of hypertension: report of the fourth working party of the British Hypertension Society. J Hum Hypertens 2004; **18:** 139–85.)

The major studies identified include the Anglo-Scandinavian Cardiac Outcomes Trial (ASCOT), the Japanese Multicenter Investigation for Cardiovascular Disease-B study (JMIC-B) and the Plaque Hypertension Lipid-Lowering Italian Study (PHYLLIS). The ASCOT is the largest of these studies, with 19,257 patients followed-up for a median of 5.5 years. This study demonstrated significantly fewer cardiovascular events and all-cause mortality among patients randomized to the amlodipine-based compared to the atenolol-based treatment. The JMIC-B and PHYLLIS are smaller studies, which reported no significant difference between ACE inhibitors versus calcium channel blockers and thiazide diuretic respectively.

Considering the data from these trials with those from earlier studies, the Guideline Development Group noted that beta-blockers were generally less effective than a comparator drug in reducing cardiovascular events, especially stroke. Hence, the group concluded that beta-blockers should *not* be used as first-line treatment of hypertension in the absence of compelling indications.

However, beta-blockers may still be considered in younger patients intolerant of ACE inhibitors or angiotensin II antagonists, of child-bearing potential (potentially teratogenic effects) and patients with high sympathetic drive. If beta-blockers are used in these patients, a calcium channel blocker (not thiazide) should be added if additional antihypertensive treatment is needed to reduce the risk of diabetes. In addition, there is no absolute need to replace beta-blockers if blood pressure is controlled (<140/90 mmHg) on a regimen which includes a beta-blocker.

The other recommendations are as outlined by the British Hypertension Society guidelines 2004. The new algorithm for the treatment of hypertension is illustrated in Figure 6.5. Beta-blockers are the obvious omission from the 2004 British Hypertension Society ABCD algorithm.

In making these recommendations, the group has also highlighted several deficiencies in the data, necessitating several assumptions. These include:

● Beta-blockers as a class, are omitted from the initial treatment algorithm although the majority of the clinical outcome data are derived from atenolol. The generalizability to other beta-blockers is not clear.

● The efficacy of thiazide diuretics is assumed to be a class effect (evidence from outcome trials for the commonly used

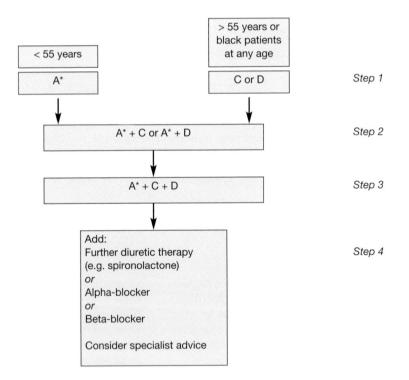

A = ACE inhibitors (*or angiotensin antagonist if ACE inhibitor intolerant), C = calcium channel blocker, D = thiazide diuretic.
Beta-blockers are not preferred initial therapy for hypertension but are an alternative to A in patients < 55 years in whom A is not tolerated or contraindicated (includes women of child-bearing potential).
Black patients are only those of African or Caribbean descent. In the absence of evidence, all other patients should be treated as non-black.

Figure 6.5
Algorithm for the treatment of hypertension (NICE update, 2006). (Adapted from National Collaborating Centre for Chronic Conditions. Hypertension: management of hypertension in adults in primary care: partial update. London: Royal College of Physicians, 2006.)

bendroflumethiazide 2.5 mg daily is lacking).

- The recommendation of ACE inhibitor (or angiotensin II antagonist) in younger patients (<55 years) is based on only limited data.

- The recommendations beyond the three-drug regime (ACE inhibitor, calcium channel blocker and thiazide diuretic) are based on general consensus, as there is little evidence to guide practice.

Further reading

Felmeden DC, Lip GYH. Antihypertensive therapy and cancer risk. *Drug Saf* 2001; **24**: 727–39.

Felmeden DC, Lip GY. Resistant hypertension and the Birmingham Hypertension Square. *Curr Hypertens Rep* 2001; **3**: 203–8.

Lip GYH, Edmunds E, Beevers DG. Should patients with hypertension receive antithrombotic therapy? *J Intern Med* 2001; **249**: 205–14.

National Collaborating Centre for Chronic Conditions. Hypertension: management of hypertension in adults in primary care: partial update. London: Royal College of Physicians, 2006.

Seventh Report of the Joint National Committee on Prevention, Detection, Evaluation and Treatment of High Blood Pressure. *Hypertension* 2003; **42**: 1206–52.

Sever PS, Poulter NR. Hypertension drug trials: past, present, and future. *J Hum Hypertens* 2000; **14**: 729–38.

Williams B, Poulter NR, Brown MJ, *et al.* Guidelines for management of hypertension: report of the fourth working party of the British Hypertension Society. *J Hum Hypertens* 2004; **18**: 139–85.

Thiazides

ALLHAT Officers and Coordinators for the ALLHAT Collaborative Research Group. Major outcomes in high-risk hypertensive patients randomized to angiotensin-converting enzyme inhibitor or calcium channel blocker vs diuretic: the Anti-hypertensive and Lipid Lowering Treatment to Prevent Heart Attack Trial (ALLHAT). *JAMA* 2002; **288**: 2981–97.

Beevers DG, Ferner RE. Why are thiazide diuretics declining in popularity? *J Hum Hypertens* 2001; **15**: 287–9.

Gosse P, Sheridan DJ, Zannad F, *et al.* Regression of left ventricular hypertrophy in hypertensive patients treated with indapamide SR 1.5 mg versus enalapril 20 mg: the LIVE study. *J Hypertens* 2000; **18**: 1465–75.

Beta-blockers

Beevers DG. Beta-blockers for hypertension: time to call a halt? *J Hum Hypertens* 1999; **12**: 807–10.

Carlberg B, Samuelsson O, Lindholm LH. Atenolol in hypertension: is it a wise choice? *Lancet* 2004; **364**: 1684–9.

Gress TW, Nieto FJ, Shahar E, *et al.* Hypertension and antihypertensive therapy as risk factors for type 2 diabetes. *N Engl J Med* 2000; **342**: 905–12.

Lindholm LH, Carlberg B, Samuelsson O. Should beta blockers remain first choice in the treatment of primary hypertension? A meta-analysis. *Lancet* 2005; **366**: 1545–53.

Messerli FH, Grossman E, Goldbourt U. Are beta-blockers efficacious as first-line therapy for hypertension in the elderly? A systematic review. *JAMA* 1998; **279**: 1903–7.

Calcium antagonists

Brown MJ, Palmer CR, Castaigne A, *et al.* Morbidity and mortality in patients randomised to double-blind treatment with a long-acting calcium-channel blocker or diuretic in the International Nifedipine GITS study: Intervention as a Goal in Hypertension Treatment (INSIGHT). *Lancet* 2000; **356**: 366–72.

Dahlof B, Sever P, Poulter NR, *et al.* Prevention of cardiovascular events with an antihypertensive regimen of amlodipine adding perindopril as required versus atenolol adding bendroflumethiazide as required, in the Anglo-Scandinavian Cardiac Outcomes Trial-Blood Pressure Lowering Arm (ASCOT-BPLA): a multicentre randomized controlled trial. *Lancet* 2005; **366**: 895–906.

Hansson L, Hedner T, Lund-Johansen P, *et al.* Randomised trial of effects of calcium antagonists compared with diuretics and beta-blockers on cardiovascular morbidity and mortality in hypertension: the Nordic Diltiazem (NORDIL) study. *Lancet* 2000; **356**: 359–65.

Hansson L, Zanchetti A, Carruthers SG, *et al.* Effects of intensive blood-pressure lowering and low-dose aspirin in patients with hypertension: principal results of the Hypertension Optimal Treatment (HOT) randomised trial. HOT Study Group. *Lancet* 1998; **351**: 1755–62.

Pahor M, Psaty BM, Alderman MH, *et al.* Health outcomes associated with calcium antagonists compared with other first-line antihypertensive therapies: a meta-analysis of randomised controlled trials. *Lancet* 2000; **356**: 1949–54.

Staessen JA, Fagard R, Thijs L, *et al.* Randomised double-blind comparison of placebo and active treatment for older patients with isolated systolic hypertension (SYST-EUR Trial). *Lancet* 1997; **350**: 754–64.

Alpha blockers

Beevers DG, Lip GY. Do alpha blockers cause heart failure and stroke? Observations from ALLHAT. *J Hum Hypertens* 2000; **14**: 287–9.

Major cardiovascular events in hypertensive patients randomized to doxazosin vs chlorthalidone: the antihypertensive and lipid-lowering treatment to prevent heart attack trial (ALLHAT). ALLHAT Collaborative Research Group. *JAMA* 2000; **283**: 1967–75.

ACE inhibitors

Abuissa H, Jones PG, Marso SP, *et al*. Angiotensin-converting enzyme inhibitors or angiotensin receptor blockers for prevention of type-2 diabetes: a meta-analysis of randomised clinical trials. *J Am Coll Cardiol* 2005; **46**: 821–6.

African American Study of Kidney Disease and Hypertension (AASK) Study Group. The effect of ramipril vs amlodipine on renal outcomes in hypertensive nephrosclerosis; a randomised controlled trial. *JAMA* 2001; **285**: 2719–28.

EUCLID Study Group. Randomised placebo-controlled trial of lisinopril in normotensive patients with diabetes and normoalbuminuria or microalbuminuria. *Lancet* 1997; **349**: 1787–92.

Fox KM. Efficacy of perindopril in reduction of cardiovascular events among patients with stable coronary artery disease: randomised, double-blind, placebo-controlled, multicentre trial (the EUROPA study). *Lancet* 2003; **362**: 782–8.

Hansson L, Lindholm LH, Niskanen L, *et al*. Effect of angiotensin-converting-enzyme inhibition compared with conventional therapy on cardiovascular morbidity and mortality in hypertension: the Captopril Prevention Project (CAPPP) randomised trial. *Lancet* 1999; **353**: 611–16.

Heart Outcomes Prevention Evaluation Study Investigators. Effects of an angiotensin-converting-enzyme inhibitor, ramipril on cardiovascular events in high-risk patients. *N Engl J Med* 2000; **342**: 145–53.

Lewis EJ, Hunsicker LG, Bain RP, *et al*. The effect of angiotensin-converting-enzyme inhibition on diabetic nephropathy. *N Engl J Med* 1993; **329**: 1456–62.

Mathew J, Sleight P, Lonn E, *et al*. Reduction of cardiovascular risk by regression of electrocardiographic markers of left ventricular hypertrophy by the angiotensin converting enzyme inhibitor, ramipril. *Circulation* 2001; **104**: 1615–21.

PEACE Trial Investigators. Angiotensin-converting-enzyme inhibition in stable coronary artery disease. *N Engl J Med* 2004; **351**: 2058–68.

PROGRESS Collaborative Group. Randomised trial of a perindopril-based blood-pressure-lowering regimen among 6,105 individuals with previous stroke or transient ischaemic attack. *Lancet* 2001; **358**: 1033–41.

Yusuf S, Sleight P, Pogue J, *et al*. Effects of an angiotensin-converting-enzyme inhibitor, ramipril on cardiovascular events in high-risk patients. The Heart Outcomes Prevention Evaluation Study Investigators. *N Engl J Med* 2000; **342**: 145–53.

Angiotensin receptor antagonists

Brenner BM, Cooper ME, de Zeeuw D, *et al*. Effects of losartan on renal and cardiovascular outcomes in patients with type 2 diabetes and nephropathy. *N Engl J Med* 2001; **345**: 861–9.

Dahlof B, Devereux RB, Kjeldsen SE, *et al*. Cardiovascular morbidity and mortality in the Losartan Intervention For Endpoint reduction in hypertension study (LIFE): a randomized trial against atenolol. *Lancet* 2002; **359**: 995–1003.

Julius S, Kjeldsen SE, Weber M, *et al*. Outcomes in hypertensive patients at high cardiovascular risk treated with regimens based on valsartan or amlodipine: the VALUE randomised trial. *Lancet* 2004; **363**: 2022–31.

Lewis EJ, Hunsicker LG, Clarke WR. Reno protective effect of the angiotensin-receptor antagonist irbesartan in patients with nephropathy due to type 2 diabetes. *N Engl J Med* 2001; **345**: 851.

Lindholm LH, Ibsen H, Dahlof B, *et al*. Cardiovascular morbidity and mortality in patients with diabetes in the Losartan Intervention For Endpoint reduction in hypertension study (LIFE): a randomized trial against atenolol. *Lancet* 2002; **359**: 1004–10.

Lithell H, Hansson L, Skoog I, *et al*. The Study of Cognition and Prognosis in the Elderly (SCOPE): principal results of a randomised double-blind intervention trial. *J Hypertens* 2003; **21**: 875–86.

Parving HH, Lehnert H, Brochner-Mortensen J, *et al*. Effect of irbesartan on the development of diabetic nephropathy in patients with type 2 diabetes. *N Engl J Med* 2001; **345**: 870–8.

Pitt B, Poole-Wilson PA, Segal R, *et al*. The effect of losartan compared with captopril on mortality in patients with symptomatic heart failure: randomised trial – the losartan heart failure survival study ELITE II. *Lancet* 2000; **355**: 1582–7.

7. Hypertension in special patient groups

Diabetes
Coronary artery disease
Cardiac failure
Hypertension following a stroke
Hypertension in the elderly
Renal disease
Peripheral vascular disease
Ethnic groups
Hyperlipidaemia
Oral contraceptives and hypertension
Hormone replacement therapy
Hypertension and anaesthesia
Hypertension in children
Metabolic syndrome

Many patients with hypertension fall into a number of special groups where there are either compelling indications from randomized controlled trials for a particular agent, or good reasons to believe that a particular agent will have favourable effects on a co-morbid condition. These 'special patient groups' are discussed here.

Diabetes

Hypertension and diabetes act synergistically to significantly increase the risk of cardiovascular mortality and morbidity, especially in association with other risk factors such as hyperlipidaemia or smoking (Figure 7.1). Hypertension is present in about a fifth of patients with insulin dependent diabetes and between 30% and 50% of patients with non-insulin dependent diabetes. This proportion may be higher (approximately two-thirds) in patients of Afro-Caribbean or Indo-Asian origin.

Patients with diabetes suffer from both macrovascular complications (e.g. myocardial infarction and peripheral vascular disease) and microvascular disease (e.g. diabetic nephropathy and retinopathy). Diabetes is also linked to an increased risk of heart failure and atrial fibrillation. These complications are further exacerbated by hypertension.

> Diabetes and hypertension combine to significantly increase the risk of vascular mortality and morbidity

In type 1 diabetes, there is clear evidence that angiotensin-converting enzyme (ACE) inhibitors reduce the progression of both retinopathy and nephropathy and possibly even neuropathy. These drugs should be regarded as first-line agents in patients with these complications.

In type 2 diabetes, lower BP targets (BP <130/80 mmHg) improve prognosis. Furthermore, reductions in proteinuria with angiotensin II antagonists, ACE inhibitors, calcium antagonists and, more recently, alpha-blockers have been noted.

Low-dose diuretics have also been found to be as effective in diabetic as non-diabetic patients. Traditionally, drugs such as thiazide diuretics have the potential to exacerbate glucose

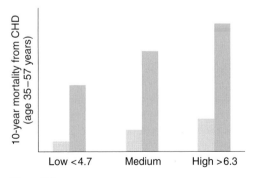

Figure 7.1
Diabetes, lipids and risk of coronary heart disease (diabetes in dark blue).

intolerance and lipid abnormalities, although these metabolic effects are minimal at low doses. However, newer diuretics such as indapamide may be more metabolically neutral. ACE inhibitors or angiotensin II receptor antagonists are probably the first choice for patients with type 2 diabetes and proteinuria, and offer special advantages by reducing the progression of diabetic nephropathy or retinopathy. Indeed, the American Diabetes Association recommends angiotensin II antagonists for patients with type 2 diabetes and proteinuria based on the wealth of clinical studies with this class of drugs (valsartan from MARVAL, losartan from RENAAL, irbesartan from IDNT and IRMA-2). The calcium antagonists and low-dose diuretics are also suitable in uncomplicated type 2 diabetes, with the aim of achieving not just 'good', but 'excellent' BP control. Beta-blockers are generally safe but non-cardioselective agents may theoretically blunt the hypoglycaemic response to insulin. As previously mentioned, beta-blockers are no longer recommended for the initial treatment of hypertension.

Hypertension in type 1 diabetes

In type 1 diabetes, an increased prevalence of hypertension is usually seen in patients with nephropathy (microalbuminuria or proteinuria); otherwise prevalence is similar to a non-diabetic population. None the less, the current British Hypertension Society guidelines regard type 1 diabetes as a high-risk population and recommend intervention with antihypertensive therapy for BP $\geq$ 140/90 mmHg. The optimal BP target of <130/80 mmHg is recommended.

In patients with type 1 diabetes, the development of hypertension may indicate the presence of the nephropathy. Certainly, BP reduction and treatment with ACE inhibitors slows the rate of renal function decline in overt diabetic nephropathy, and delays progression from the microalbuminuric phase to overt nephropathy. These drugs might have a specific renoprotective action in patients with incipient or overt nephropathy and are to be

recommended as first-line therapy. The data for angiotensin II receptor antagonists in type 1 diabetes are scantier and therefore they cannot be regarded as first-line therapy over ACE inhibitors. Indeed, type 1 diabetes with nephropathy represents a compelling indication for ACE inhibitor therapy.

For renoprotection, BP control is crucial, and recommended BP targets should be achieved by multiple drug therapy.

The threshold for antihypertensive treatment in type 1 diabetes with nephropathy is BP $\geq$ 140/90 mmHg, aiming for a target BP <130/80 mmHg, or even lower (BP <125/75 mmHg) if there is proteinuria $\geq$ 1 g every 24 hours. If persistent microalbuminuria or proteinuria is present, these patients may also benefit from ACE inhibitors or angiotensin receptor antagonists, even if BP is normal. As is evident from the recent HOPE trial, the beneficial effects of ACE inhibition (ramipril in the HOPE trial) are independent of the degree of BP reduction (Figure 7.2). In view of the high cardiovascular risk, statin and aspirin therapy are also recommended, the latter when BP is adequately controlled (<150/90 mmHg).

Hypertension in type 2 diabetes

Hypertension is very common in type 2 diabetes, and these patients are frequently obese. In type 2 diabetes, hypertension is prevalent in over 70% of patients and may even precede the onset of diabetes. The presence of hypertension in type 2 diabetes is highly predictive of cardiovascular and microvascular complications, with an overall 10-year cardiovascular event rate of >30%. These are predominantly coronary events.

The threshold for intervention with antihypertensive therapy is BP $\geq$ 140/90 mmHg in type 2 diabetes, irrespective of other risk factors. In the UKPDS (United Kingdom Prospective Diabetes Study), antihypertensive therapy was the only intervention that

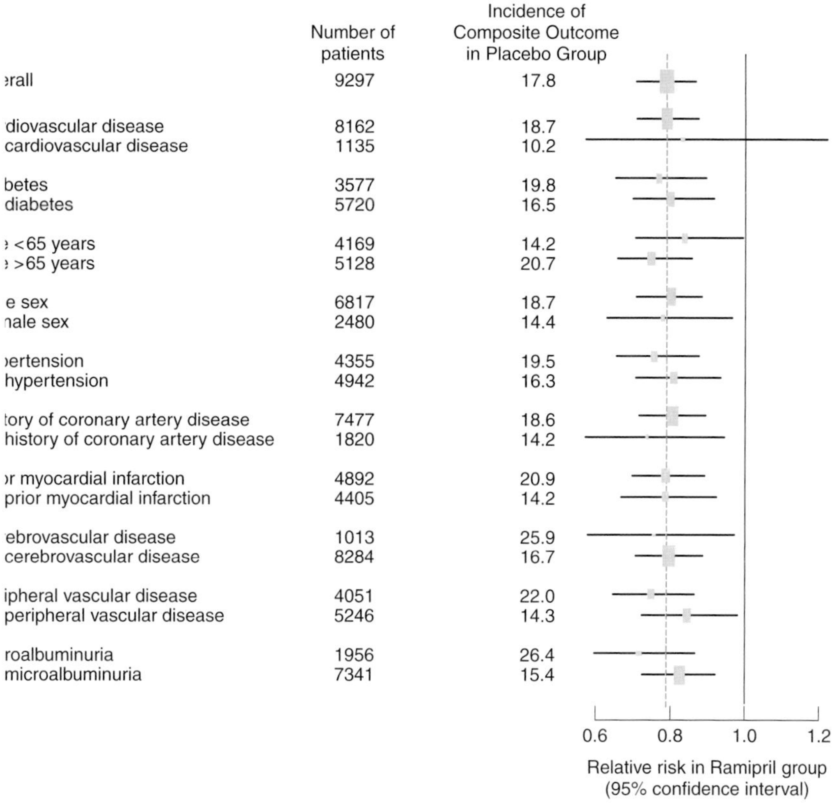

	Number of patients	Incidence of Composite Outcome in Placebo Group	
?rall	9297	17.8	
diovascular disease	8162	18.7	
cardiovascular disease	1135	10.2	
betes	3577	19.8	
diabetes	5720	16.5	
? <65 years	4169	14.2	
? >65 years	5128	20.7	
e sex	6817	18.7	
nale sex	2480	14.4	
?ertension	4355	19.5	
hypertension	4942	16.3	
tory of coronary artery disease	7477	18.6	
history of coronary artery disease	1820	14.2	
?r myocardial infarction	4892	20.9	
prior myocardial infarction	4405	14.2	
ebrovascular disease	1013	25.9	
cerebrovascular disease	8284	16.7	
ipheral vascular disease	4051	22.0	
peripheral vascular disease	5246	14.3	
roalbuminuria	1956	26.4	
microalbuminuria	7341	15.4	

0.6   0.8   1.0   1.2

Relative risk in Ramipril group
(95% confidence interval)

Figure 7.2
The benefit of ACE inhibition is consistent across various subgroups, including patients without a history of hypertension. (Adapted from Yusuf et al. N Engl J Med 2000; **342**: 145–53.)

decreased mortality rates in patients with type 2 diabetes and proved more effective than tight glycaemic control in protecting against microvascular and macrovascular disease.

In UKPDS, patients with hypertension and type 2 diabetes assigned to tight control of blood pressure, with captopril or atenolol, achieved a significant reduction in risk of 24% for any endpoints related to diabetes and 37% for microvascular disease. In comparison, intensive blood glucose control in the UK prospective diabetes study decreased the risk of any diabetes-related endpoint by 12% (P=0.029) and microvascular disease by 25% (P=0.0099). Those in the Hypertension Optimal Trial (HOT) and the elderly diabetics with isolated systolic hypertension from the Syst-Eur trial also showed marked benefits after receiving treatment, with a BP target <140/80 mmHg. Specifically, diabetic patients in the HOT study had a 51% reduction in major cardiovascular events in the target group with a diastolic pressure <80 mmHg compared to the group with a target diastolic pressure of <90 mmHg.

In the Irbesartan Diabetic Nephropathy Trial (IDNT), the angiotensin II receptor antagonist irbesartan was compared with amlodipine and with placebo in diabetic patients with overt proteinuria. Both drugs reduced the blood pressure by roughly equal amounts but only irbesartan caused any delay in the progression of diabetic nephropathy.

In the IRbesartan MicroAlbuminuria Type 2 Diabetes Mellitus in Hypertensive patients (IRMA-2) study, irbesartan at two different dose levels (150 mg and 300 mg daily) was compared with placebo in diabetic patients who had microproteinuria. This trial was able to demonstrate a statistically significant dose–response curve, with the 300 mg dose of irbesartan being more effective than 150 mg at reducing microproteinuria or normalizing albumen excretion.

The third study, the Reduction of Endpoints in Non-Insulin Dependent Diabetes Mellitus with the Angiotensin II Antagonist Losartan (RENAAL) trial, losartan was compared with placebo in patients with overt diabetic nephropathy. This trial was able to demonstrate a 16% reduction in the doubling of serum creatinine and a 28% reduction in end-stage renal disease (Figure 7.3). Another finding which was considered as a secondary endpoint was a 32% reduction in hospitalization for heart failure (Figure 7.4).

Suggested drug treatment

The choice of first-line drug for type 2 diabetes favours angiotensin II antagonists and ACE inhibitors (as first-line), with the addition of dihydropyridine calcium antagonists and low-dose thiazide diuretics to achieve target blood pressures. The UKPDS study suggested that regimens based on ACE inhibition (captopril) and beta-blockade (atenolol) were equally effective at reducing macrovascular complications, but the treatment groups were too small to exclude this difference.

In type 2 diabetic subjects with nephropathy, hypertension accelerates the decline of renal function, which is slowed by treatment with antihypertensive therapy. While the ACE inhibitors and angiotensin II receptor antagonists have an antiproteinuric action and delay the progression from microalbuminuria to overt nephropathy, it is less clear whether they have specific renoprotective action beyond BP reduction in overt nephropathy complicating type 2 diabetes. As for patients with type 1 diabetes, statin and aspirin therapy should be offered to all patients with type 2 diabetes and hypertension, as they are considered to be at high cardiovascular disease (CVD) risk.

Coronary artery disease

Hypertension is a risk factor for the development of atheromatous coronary artery

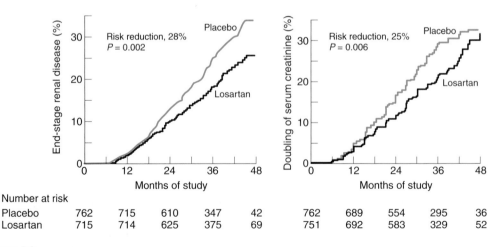

Figure 7.3
The RENAAL study. (Adapted from Brenner *et al.* N Engl J Med 2001; **345**: 861–9.)

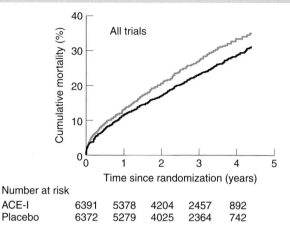

Figure 7.4
A secondary endpoint in the RENAAL study. (Adapted from Brenner *et al*. *N Engl J Med* 2001; **345**: 861–9.)

disease. Coronary artery disease (CAD), as manifest by angina and myocardial infarction, is more common in patients with hypertension. There appears to be an almost 'dose–response' relationship between coronary risk and increasing BP. While angina usually results from coronary artery atherosclerosis, it can also result from relative ischaemia in severe left ventricular hypertrophy (LVH). In any case, hypertensive patients with overt coronary artery disease are at particularly high risk of further cardiac events. In the peri-infarction state, BP may have fallen so that the diagnosis of hypertension may be missed and only become apparent at subsequent outpatient clinic visits.

Suggested drug treatment

Effective treatment of hypertension may improve the symptoms of angina, regardless of the drugs used. As beta-blockers are useful for secondary prevention after myocardial infarction, they are the first-choice drugs for hypertensive patients who have sustained a myocardial infarct. If beta-blockers are contraindicated, non-dihydropyridine calcium antagonists (e.g. verapamil or diltiazem) may be beneficial provided there is no evidence of

heart failure or left ventricular dysfunction. Verapamil should not be given with a beta-blocker as it can result in asystole, heart block or cardiac failure.

> Beta-blockers are the first-choice drug to treat angina symptoms in hypertensive patients

There is some evidence that diltiazem may be beneficial following non-Q-wave myocardial infarction. The dihydropyridine calcium antagonists (particularly nifedipine) should be avoided both in the immediate period post-infarction and in unstable angina. Short-acting dihydropyridine calcium antagonists (e.g. immediate-release nifedipine) may also exacerbate angina by promoting reflex tachycardia. The presence of heart failure or left ventricular dysfunction post-myocardial infarction is a strong indication for ACE inhibitor therapy.

Patients taking thiazide diuretics who are admitted with myocardial infarction should have their serum potassium concentrations checked; they may have hypokalaemia, which can exacerbate the tendency to cardiac arrhythmia and sudden death.

Cardiac failure

Usually heart failure develops in the hypertensive patient in association with coronary artery disease. Rarely, severe hypertension can be associated with heart failure. Echocardiography can help diagnose structural heart disease and assess cardiac function.

Suggested drug treatment

Many trials have firmly established the role of ACE inhibitors in patients with heart failure and asymptomatic left ventricular dysfunction (Figure 7.5), and the benefits are greater with more severe heart failure. Many such patients have coexisting hypertension. Caution is needed in the use of verapamil or diltiazem for hypertension in patients with heart failure. Long-acting dihydropyridine calcium channel blockers have neutral effect with regard to mortality in heart failure due to systolic dysfunction.

Recent data support the use of angiotensin II receptor antagonists as an alternative to the ACE inhibitors (in ACE inhibitor intolerant patients). Initial subgroup analysis of the Val-HeFT (valsartan) trial suggested potential

adverse effects with the then so-called 'triple therapy' – the addition of angiotensin II antagonist to ACE inhibitors and beta-blockers. However, this has now been refuted by the more recent (and robust) data from CHARM (candesartan), which suggests modest but significant benefit in patients with heart failure secondary to left ventricular systolic dysfunction. Angiotensin II antagonists should therefore be used in ACE inhibitor intolerant patients. The combination of hydralazine and nitrates may be used if ACE inhibitors (and angiotensin II antagonist) are contraindicated or cause side-effects, although this regimen may be better than ACE inhibitors for Afro-Caribbean hypertension patients with heart failure.

In stable patients with chronic heart failure, a beta-blocker (e.g. carvedilol, bisoprolol or nebivolol) added to ACE inhibitors and diuretics has a beneficial effect on mortality and morbidity. Beta-blockers should be initiated in patients with heart failure under specialist advice. Transient deterioration in heart failure symptoms may occur with beta-blocker therapy, and should therefore be started at low-dose and uptitrated slowly ('go low, go slow'). Like ACE inhibitors, beta-blockers are recommended in patients with asymptomatic left ventricular dysfunction.

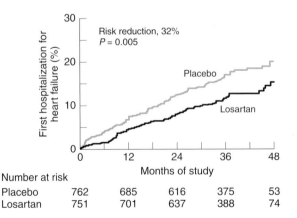

Figure 7.5
Meta-analysis of clinical studies confirms the benefit of ACE inhibitors in heart failure due to left ventricular dysfunction. (Adapted from *Flather et al. Lancet* 2000; **355**: 1575–81.)

Additional blockade of the renin–angiotensin–aldosterone system with the aldosterone antagonist spironolactone also significantly reduces mortality and morbidity in patients established on standard therapy (including the ACE inhibitors) (Figure 7.6). Eplerenone, another aldosterone antagonist, has also been shown to improve clinical outcome when introduced early in patients with post-MI heart failure. Close monitoring of electrolytes is mandatory as the use of spironolactone or eplerenone with ACE inhibitors may lead to dangerous hyperkalaemia.

Hypertension following a stroke

Uncontrolled hypertension in association with cerebrovascular disease is a risk factor for further cerebrovascular events. It is nevertheless unclear whether or not the treatment of mild hypertension post-stroke is of benefit, especially as in the immediate post-stroke period, cerebral blood flow autoregulation is disordered so that rapid reductions in BP can reduce cerebral perfusion and even cause stroke extension. Recent data from the Perindopril pROtection aGainst REcurrent Stroke Study (PROGRESS) trial suggest that treatment with ACE inhibitors in patients who have had a previous (non-acute) stroke significantly reduced mortality and cardiovascular morbidity. In this study, 6105 hypertensive and non-hypertensive patients who had had stroke (haemorrhagic or ischaemic) or transient ischaemic attack (TIA) with no major disability within the past five years, were randomized to perindopril 4 mg daily, with indapamide (2.5 mg daily) added at the

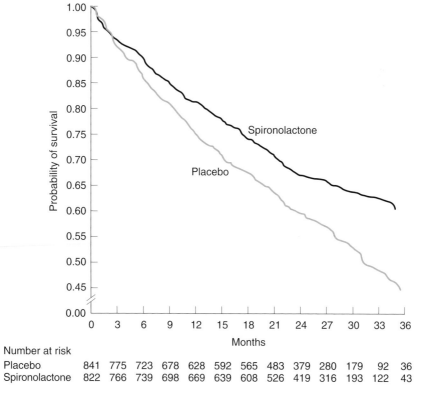

Figure 7.6
Spironolactone reduces mortality in the RALES study. (Adapted from Pitt *et al. N Engl J Med* 1999; **341**: 709–17.)

discretion of the treating physician; or matched placebo. After four years of follow-up, active treatment (60% received both drugs, while 40% received perindopril alone) reduced BP by 9/4 mmHg and stroke recurrence by 28% compared to placebo and that of major cardiovascular complications by 26%. In the subgroup of active treatment patients who received both perindopril and indapamide, BP was reduced by 12/5 mmHg, and the risk of stroke was reduced by 43%. Single-drug therapy with perindopril alone reduced BP by 5/3 mmHg, but produced no significant reduction in the risk of stroke.

In cerebral infarction, low-dose aspirin (75–300 mg) should also be prescribed, although if atrial fibrillation is present warfarin should be considered.

The role of antihypertensive medication during an acute stroke is controversial. Blood pressure is often elevated during the stroke period and this is regarded as a compensatory physiological response to maintain cerebral perfusion. As a result, it is common practice to reduce or withhold antihypertensive treatment. However,

if the BP persistently exceeds 180/110 mmHg, then nifedipine (slow-release) 10–20 mg tablets or 25 mg atenolol may be prescribed with the aim of reducing BP cautiously by 10–15%.

Hypertension in the elderly

It was a widely and incorrectly held myth that a rise in BP with age was inevitable and harmless, and that isolated systolic hypertension was of no consequence. The elderly have a higher prevalence of isolated systolic hypertension (defined as BP ≥ 160/<90 mmHg), occurring in >50% of people over 60 years of age. Systolic BP also rises steadily with age. These elderly hypertensive patients have a high risk of cardiovascular complications when compared to younger patients. Treatment with antihypertensive therapy reduces this risk, particularly in very high-risk groups, such as elderly patients with type 2 diabetes and hypertension. Treatment has been shown to reduce heart failure by 50% and possibly reduce dementia (Figure 7.7).

Evidence exists that patients aged up to at least 80 years benefit from antihypertensive treatment.

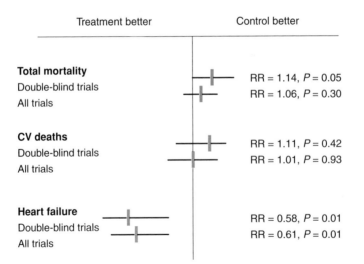

Figure 7.7
Anti-hypertensive treatment effects on cardiovascular outcomes in the elderly. (Adapted from Gueyffier *et al. Lancet* 1999; **353**: 793–6.)

Newly diagnosed hypertension patients aged 80 years or more should be considered for treatment provided they are generally fit and have a reasonable life expectancy.

In the very frail elderly, assessment of the risk:benefit ratio is recommended. One ongoing trial, the Hypertension in the Very Elderly Trial (HYVET), will provide data on treating hypertension in patients aged >80 years. This is likely to be the last placebo-controlled trial and is a double blind study of over 2000 hypertensive patients aged over 80 years. The primary endpoint is stroke events (fatal and non-fatal) and the trial is powered to determine whether there is a 35% reduction in total stroke events between placebo and active treatment. Treatment consists of a diuretic (indapamide SR 1.5 mg daily) and additional ACE inhibitor (perindopril) if required, with a five-year average follow-up. Secondary endpoints include total mortality, cardiovascular mortality, cardiac mortality, stroke mortality and skeletal fracture.

> The elderly are more likely to have isolated systolic hypertension

Elderly hypertensive patients respond to non-pharmacological measures to lower BP as well as younger patients. In a trial of non-pharmacological interventions in the elderly (TONE), reducing sodium intake to less than 2 g/day reduced BP over 30 months and about 40% of those on low-salt diet were able to discontinue their antihypertensive treatment. Low-dose thiazide diuretics and long-acting dihydropyridine calcium antagonists should be considered as first-line drugs for the treatment of hypertension. Beta-blockers are less effective than thiazides as first-line treatment and meta-analyses suggest that beta-blockers decrease stroke but no other cardiovascular events in the elderly. However, the elderly have more co-morbidity and may be open to more polypharmacy and drug interactions. Postural hypotension, defined as a drop in systolic and diastolic BP of > 20 and 10 mmHg respectively,

is more common in the elderly and periodic assessment of lying and standing BP is recommended. Overall, however, the concern that the elderly tolerate antihypertensive drugs poorly is probably exaggerated.

Renal disease

Renovascular disease (renal artery stenosis)

Renovascular disease (renal artery stenosis) is relatively uncommon, but is probably the most frequent curable cause of hypertension. ACE inhibitors may cause or worsen renal impairment in patients with critical renovascular disease. For this reason, they should be used with caution in patients with advanced chronic renal impairment, preferably with specialist supervision.

Clues suggesting renovascular disease are:

● onset of hypertension before the age of 30
● documented sudden onset, or recent worsening, of hypertension in middle age
● accelerated (malignant) hypertension
● resistant hypertension (to a three-drug regimen)
● renal impairment of unknown cause
● elevation of serum creatinine by ACE inhibitor or angiotensin II antagonist treatment
● peripheral vascular disease or severe generalized atherosclerotic disease
● recurrent pulmonary oedema or heart failure with no obvious cause.

Patients with any of these features should be referred for specialist advice because the investigations required to confirm or exclude renovascular disease are complex.

Renal failure

Many patients with renal failure have hypertension, but whether or not the hypertension is the cause of renal failure, or is secondary to it, often remains unclear.

Hypertensive patients with elevated serum creatinine or proteinuria may have parenchymal or obstructive renal disease, and should be referred for specialist evaluation.

Accelerated (malignant) hypertension requires immediate hospital treatment because it causes rapid loss of renal function, which can be irreversible if untreated. Otherwise, there is little evidence that non-malignant essential hypertension causes renal failure. The corollary is that renal impairment, in the absence of previous accelerated phase hypertension, suggests primary renal disease or renovascular disease. In patients with chronic renal impairment, hypertension accelerates the rate of loss of renal function and good BP control is essential to retard this process.

Hypertension treatment in renal failure

Effective treatment of hypertension slows the progression of renal failure. Meta-analysis of all controlled trials showed a 30% reduction in incidence of end-stage renal failure with ACE inhibitors, which may not all be explained by BP reduction alone. ACE inhibitors are renoprotective and delay the progression of both diabetic and non-diabetic nephropathy. Angiotensin receptor antagonists have also been shown to reduce proteinuria and may be a suitable alternative to ACE inhibitors, especially in (type 2) diabetic nephropathy. Hence, ACE inhibitors should be the drugs of first choice for patients with renal disease except in those with bilateral renal artery stenosis (or stenosis in the artery to a single kidney).

The optimal BP should be lower (BP <125/75 mmHg) in patients with renal disease and proteinuria >1 g/24 hours. This lower BP target means that multiple antihypertensive agents are needed in most patients. Thiazide diuretics may be ineffective in patients with renal impairment and loop diuretics (i.e. furosemide), often in high-doses, are frequently required. Calcium channel blockers and alpha-blockers are useful additional agents. The dose of renally excreted antihypertensive drugs may

need to be adjusted. Of note, patients with impaired renal function are particularly salt-sensitive, and dietary salt reduction is important. In addition, patients with renal failure have a very high risk of cardiovascular complications, and may benefit from aspirin or statin treatment in addition to non-pharmacological measures to reduce their cardiovascular risk (Figure 7.8).

Peripheral vascular disease

Hypertension is a common and important risk factor for vascular disorders, including peripheral vascular disease (PVD). Intermittent claudication is the most common symptomatic manifestation of PVD. It is also an important predictor of cardiovascular death, increasing it by three-fold, and increasing all-cause mortality two- to five-fold. Of hypertensive patients at presentation, about 2–5% have intermittent claudication, and this increases with age. Similarly, 35–55% of patients with PVD at presentation also have hypertension. Patients who suffer from hypertension with PVD have a greatly increased risk of myocardial infarction and stroke. Apart from the epidemiological associations, hypertension contributes to the pathogenesis of atherosclerosis, the basic pathological process underlying PVD. Peripheral vascular disease is exacerbated by increases in serum lipid concentrations and by smoking.

> Hypertension is found in one-third to one-half of patients with PVD, and patients with both have a much greater risk of suffering strokes or myocardial infarction

Treatment of hypertension in patients with peripheral vascular disease

None of the large antihypertensive treatment trials have adequately addressed whether or not a reduction in BP causes a decrease in PVD incidence. Treatment of hypertension in patients with PVD should follow the conventional treatment algorithm outlined in the previous chapter. However, ACE inhibitors should be used

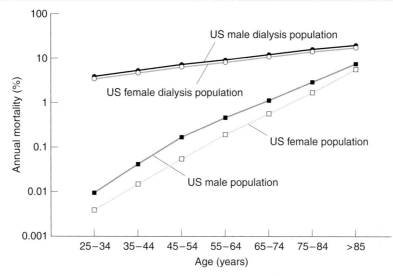

Figure 7.8
Cardiovascular mortality in dialysis patients. (Adapted from *Lancet* 2000; **356**: 147–52.)

with caution as there may be undiagnosed atheromatous renal artery stenosis (see above). In patients with peripheral vascular disease, an 'exquisite' or over-rapid fall in BP in response to ACE inhibitor, or a significant rise in serum creatinine levels, raises a strong possibility of underlying renal artery stenosis. Vasodilators, e.g. calcium antagonists and alpha-blockers, are useful agents in such patients. Calcium channel blockers may modestly improve the symptoms of claudication. There is the misconception that beta-blockers may worsen peripheral vascular disease, but trials comparing beta-blockers with a placebo did not significantly influence claudication distance. Nevertheless, they should be avoided in patients with rest pain or gangrene.

Ethnic groups

The ethnic differences in the incidence, pathophysiology and management of hypertension are particularly pertinent to the Afro-Caribbean population, who have a high prevalence of hypertension and associated complications such as strokes and renal impairment. The lack of large, long-term prospective randomized trials with hard

outcome data has made it difficult to ascertain the precise benefits for the different antihypertensive agents in specific ethnic groups. There is also the difficulty of defining a solely Afro-Caribbean or white population, as many subgroups may exist within a particular ethnic group.

There are clear ethnic differences in cardiovascular disease (CVD) and its risk factors. Despite an increased prevalence of both hypertension and diabetes, the overall risk of coronary artery disease (CAD) in the Afro-Caribbean male population in Europe, in the Caribbean and to a lesser extent in North America, is lower than in white males. By contrast, Indo-Asians have an excess prevalence of CAD. This contrast may be due to a multitude of reasons, and some suggest that the traditional risk factors do not fully explain the ethnic differences in CVD and stroke.

> Ethnic differences are important in how hypertension is managed (especially in Afro-Caribbean people), and also for the risk factors associated with CVD

Afro-Caribbeans

Hypertension is known to occur more frequently in the Afro-Caribbean population and is associated with a higher incidence of cerebrovascular and renal complications. Strokes are more common and hypertension-associated end-stage renal failure is up to 20 times more frequent in Afro-Caribbean patients than in non-Afro-Caribbean patients.

In addition, there is a greater tendency to develop LVH, and Afro-Caribbean patients with mild hypertension have a two-fold higher prevalence of LVH compared to non-Afro-Caribbeans with comparable BP levels. In the West Birmingham malignant hypertension register, there was an excess of Afro-Caribbean patients with malignant hypertension, higher BP and more severe renal impairment at presentation; these patients had a worse overall median survival rate and an increased rate of progression to dialysis. Therefore, Afro-Caribbean patients with malignant hypertension did not do worse simply because they were Afro-Caribbean, but appeared to have poorer BP control and more complications such as renal damage.

> Afro-Caribbean patients are 20 times more likely to develop hypertension-associated end-stage renal failure than white patients

Afro-Caribbean patients with hypertension exhibit enhanced sodium retention with a higher incidence of salt-sensitive hypertension, expanded plasma volume and a higher prevalence of low plasma renin activity. For this reason, hypertension in Afro-Caribbeans is often sensitive to dietary salt restriction. In patients with no evidence of target organ damage, a low salt diet may occasionally be sufficient to control BP. Reduced sodium-potassium ATPase activity is also associated with hypertension in Afro-Caribbean patients, combined with a tendency towards increased intracellular sodium and calcium concentrations. In addition, proteinuria has been observed more frequently in African-Americans compared to white patients with similar creatinine levels. Control of dietary sodium should be combined with other non-pharmacological measures including weight control, alcohol moderation and regular exercise.

Use of drugs acting on the renin–angiotensin system

Afro-Caribbean patients tend to have lower levels of renin than white patients (Figure 7.9) and tend to respond less well to drugs that act on the renin–angiotensin system, such as beta-blockers, ACE inhibitors and angiotensin II antagonists. In contrast, these patients respond well to calcium antagonists, alpha-blockers and diuretics. Where there are clear indications for these agents, such as post-myocardial infarction or heart failure, these patients should not be denied ACE inhibitors and beta-blockers. Indeed, Afro-Caribbean patients may respond to ACE-inhibition or beta-blockade given in combination with drugs that activate the renin–angiotensin system, i.e. diuretics, calcium channel blockers or alpha-blockers. Of note, angioedema is more common with the use of ACE inhibitors in the Afro-Caribbean population.

South Asians

South Asians (from the Indian subcontinent) have a high prevalence of hypertension, obesity, insulin resistance and type 2 diabetes, giving

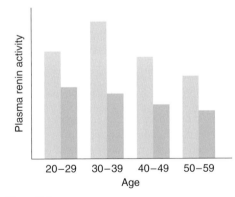

Figure 7.9
Plasma renin in Afro-Caribbean (in dark blue) and Caucasian patients with hypertension.

rise to the so-called 'metabolic syndrome'. This ethnic group is at particularly high risk of CHD. The response to antihypertensive drug treatment in South Asian patients is similar to that in white Europeans although data are limited. Good control of BP is particularly important in those with diabetes, and aspirin and/or statin treatment may be indicated for those at high risk of CHD.

Hyperlipidaemia

The best strategy for patients at high cardiovascular risk with hyperlipidaemia and hypertension is to treat both with different drugs, and not worry too much about small changes in cholesterol. In patients at high risk of CVD, HMG coenzyme A inhibitors (statins) have been shown to reduce cardiovascular events. As the beta-blockers and high-dose diuretics aggravate hyperlipidaemia, they should be avoided in people whose hyperlipidaemia is difficult to control. However, in reality, the clinical effect of these drugs on lipids is small.

Oral contraceptives and hypertension

The combined oral contraceptives (OCs) have a small adverse effect on BP – approximately 5/3 mmHg. The Nurses' Health Study found that current users of OCs had a small but significantly increased risk of hypertension compared to never users. Controlled studies suggest a return of BP to pre-treatment levels within three months of discontinuation, indicating that the BP effect is reversible.

However, the increase in BP may also be idiosyncratic and may occur many months or years after first using a combined OC. In a small proportion of women (approximately 1%) severe hypertension may be induced. As the BP response to any combined OC preparation is unpredictable, and there is a small increase in cardiovascular risk associated with OC use, BP should certainly be measured before starting OC use and then every six months thereafter. It

should not be forgotten that OCs can increase the risk of venous thromboembolism.

If other risk factors for cardiovascular disease (e.g. smoking or migraine) exist, other non-hormonal forms of contraception should be sought. In those women for whom other methods of contraception are unacceptable, careful monitoring of BP is recommended. Antihypertensive therapy should be considered if BP remains elevated.

> Oral contraceptives can affect hypertension slightly although in some cases hypertension can be severe

Hormone replacement therapy

For many years, hormone replacement therapy (HRT) was considered to be contraindicated in postmenopausal women with hypertension. Many such women were excluded from HRT because of concerns that HRT might have an adverse effect on BP. This perception was mainly due to the effects of oral contraceptive drugs, especially the oestrogen component, in increasing BP. Differences exist between the formulation and doses of oestrogen preparations used either as oral contraceptives in premenopausal women (in whom high-dose synthetic oestrogens are used) or as HRT in postmenopausal women (in whom low 'replacement' doses of natural oestrogens are used). This is not inconsequential, as postmenopausal women represent the largest category of women at risk of hypertension.

The Women's Health Initiative, the largest longitudinal study to evaluate the effect of HRT on BP, found an average of 1 mmHg increase in systolic BP over 5.6 years of follow-up among patients randomized to conjugated oestrogen and medroxyprogesterone compared to placebo. This study contrasts with the results of other smaller studies. Overall, the effect of HRT on BP is likely to be modest. However, the question of HRT and BP may be of little clinical relevance in view of the recent reports of adverse cardiovascular outcome associated with the use of HRT and the already well-documented risk of venous thromboembolism.

> The question of hormone replacement therapy and blood pressure may be of little clinical relevance in view of the recent reports of adverse cardiovascular outcome associated with the use of HRT

Treating hypertension in conjunction with hormone replacement therapy

HRT is certainly not contraindicated for women with hypertension. Women with hypertension should not be denied access to HRT as long as BP levels can be controlled by antihypertensive medication. In view of the lack of consensus in the prescribing habits of HRT, suitable guidelines are as follows:

- All clinicians should measure BP before starting HRT.
- In normotensive postmenopausal women, BP should be measured annually following the start of HRT. One exception may be the use of premarin, where a follow-up BP measurement should probably be made at three months (in view of reports of a possible rare idiosyncratic rise in BP).
- In hypertensive menopausal women, BP should at least be measured initially and at six-monthly intervals thereafter. If BP is labile or difficult to control, three-monthly measurements should be taken. If a hypertensive woman on HRT demonstrates a rise in BP, careful monitoring or observation and perhaps an alteration or increase of their antihypertensive treatment should be considered.

Hypertension and anaesthesia

The issues regarding hypertension and anaesthesia can be related to the evaluation of the BP itself (preoperative) and the use of antihypertensive agents (intra- and postoperative). Many non-urgent surgical procedures are postponed unnecessarily when patients are erroneously diagnosed as hypertensive. In fact they are simply exhibiting anxiety-related white-coat hypertension caused by admission to hospital.

Criteria for anaesthesia in the hypertensive patient

If the patient has mild asymptomatic hypertension with no target organ damage, and is otherwise fit and well, then he/she is at no particular risk in the perioperative period. In contrast, patients with severe hypertension, especially those with target organ damage, are at risk of perioperative complications (including arrhythmias or myocardial infarction). If BP >180/110, elective surgery should be postponed in these patients until they have been fully assessed and better BP control has been achieved. Parenteral control of hypertension is rarely needed because patients are usually on bed rest and receiving opioid analgesia, which reduce BP.

Suspension of hypertensive medication before anaesthesia

Care is needed in those patients taking particular antihypertensive drugs as some anaesthetic agents may have a hypotensive effect. The ACE inhibitors may block the response of the renin–angiotensin system, resulting in hypotension following blood loss, while the beta-blockers may block the compensatory rise in heart rate associated with fluid loss. However, beta-blockers should not be stopped in the perioperative period because this class of drug has benefits in preventing postoperative arrhythmias, e.g. including atrial fibrillation. In patients with coronary artery disease, stopping the beta-blocker may provoke myocardial ischaemia. In those cases where antihypertensive drugs have to be stopped, they should be started again as soon as practically possible.

Hypertension in children

Hypertension is a rare problem in children and, where present, it is usually the result of another condition (possibly renal or vasculitic diseases). Children with systemic illness should have their BP checked. It is possible that the origin of adult essential hypertension starts in childhood or even infancy. Children whose BP exceeds the 90th percentile for their age need careful rechecking, and if they exceed the 95th percentile, referral to hospital specialists and detailed investigation is mandatory.

> In children, hypertension is often a symptom of another condition

Measuring BP in children

It is not considered justifiable to screen BP in all children. Children with an initial high BP tend to show a faster rise with advancing age, especially when obese. Under the age of three years, BP measurement can only be achieved with Doppler flow equipment. BP should be measured with the child in a comfortable sitting position (although infants may be supine), with the right arm exposed and supported at the heart level and an appropriate-sized cuff used. However, phase V sounds may be difficult to obtain in children. The guidelines therefore accept the Korotkoff sounds of K4 diastolic BP in the standards for infants and children aged from three years to 12 years, and K5 diastolic BP for adolescents aged from 13 to 18. The

fourth and fifth Korotkoff diastolic sounds should still be recorded if both are heard.

Treatment of hypertension in children

As with general management of hypertension, non-pharmacological therapy should be initiated along with salt restriction and diet control. Beta-blockers, calcium antagonists and alpha-blockers are generally safe for use by children. However, thiazides theoretically have long-term metabolic effects and so are best avoided in children. The ACE inhibitors should also be used with caution in children with renal disease.

Metabolic syndrome

Metabolic syndrome describes the frequent coalition of multiple cardiovascular risk factors – abdominal obesity, hypertension, abnormal glucose tolerance (impaired fasting glucose, impaired glucose tolerance or diabetes) and dyslipidaemia (high triglyceride and low HDL cholesterol levels). The World Health Organization and Adult Treatment Panel (ATP)-III diagnostic criteria for metabolic syndrome are summarized in Table 7.1. Metabolic syndrome diagnosed by either of these criteria identifies patients at increased risk of diabetes, CVD and all-cause mortality. The International Diabetes Federation diagnostic criteria build on the ATP-III criteria and include ethnic-specific values for waist circumference (Table 7.2).

Table 7.1
Definition of metabolic syndrome

NCEP definition	WHO definition
At least three of the following: • Fasting plasma glucose >6.1 mmol/L • Waist girth >102 cm (men), >88 cm (women) • Serum triglycerides ≥ 1.7 mmol/L • Serum HDL <1.0 mmol/L (men), <1.3 mmol/L (women) • Blood pressure ≥ 130/85 mmHg	Insulin resistance, impaired glucose regulation or diabetes AND at least two of the following: • Hypertension (blood pressure 140/90 mmHg) • Central obesity (waist–hip ratio 0.9 in men, 0.85 in women or BMI >30 kg/m²) • Dyslipidaemia (serum triglyceride >1.7 mmol/L or HDL <0.9 in men and <1.0 in women) • Microalbuminuria (urine albumin excretion rate ≥ 20 µg/min)

NCEP, National Cholesterol Education Program; WHO, World Health Organization; HDL, high-density lipoprotein; BMI, body mass index.

Table 7.2
International Diabetes Federation definition of metabolic syndrome

- Central obesity
- Waist circumference – ethnic-specific (*see below*)*

Plus any two of the following:
- Raised triglycerides
  >1.7 mmol/L (or specific treatment of this abnormality)
- Reduced HDL cholesterol
  <1.03 mmol/L in men, <1.29 mmol/L in women (or specific treatment of this abnormality)
- Raised blood pressure
  Systolic ≥ 130 mmHg
  Diastolic ≥ 85 mmHg
  (or treatment of previous hypertension)
- Raised fasting plasma glucose
  >5.6 mmol/L or previously diagnosed type 2 diabetes

(glucose tolerance test recommended if fasting glucose >5.6 mmol/L but not required to define this syndrome)

*Ethnic groups
Europids – Men ≥ 94 cm, Women ≥ 80 cm
South Asians – Men ≥ 90 cm, Women ≥ 80 cm
Chinese – Men ≥ 90 cm, Women ≥ 80 cm
Japanese – Men ≥ 85 cm, Women ≥ 90 cm
Ethnic South and Central Americans – Men ≥ 90 cm, Women ≥ 80 cm
Sub-Saharan Africans – Men ≥ 94 cm, Women ≥ 80 cm
Eastern Mediterranean and Middle East populations – Men ≥ 94 cm, Women ≥ 80 cm

Treatment

Lifestyle changes, with the aim of halting weight gain or encouraging healthy weight loss, are the cornerstone for the clinical management of people with metabolic syndrome (see Chapter 6: Non-pharmacological management). Pharmacological adjuncts may be tried, especially in people with clear motivation and in conjunction with appropriate advice, support and counselling, to facilitate weight loss. The National Institute of Clinical Excellence (NICE) guidelines support the use of orlistat (a lipase inhibitor) for people who have lost at least 2.5 kg in weight by non-pharmacological

measures. The novel endocannabinoid receptor antagonist rimonabant has been shown to lower blood pressure and reverse the metabolic abnormalities associated with the metabolic syndrome. Sibutramine, which has an adverse effect on BP, is not recommended in hypertension.

Other cardiovascular risk factors should also be addressed in a multifactorial approach to the management of metabolic syndrome. Blood pressure targets are as outlined previously (see Chapter 6). As patients with metabolic syndrome have an increased risk of developing diabetes, beta-blockers and thiazide diuretics (and especially their combination) are generally not advisable as first-line agents. In contrast, ACE inhibitors and angiotensin II antagonists may be considered as first-line antihypertensive therapy in patients with metabolic syndrome as several clinical trials have shown them to reduce new-onset diabetes.

The Joint British Societies guidelines recommend statin therapy for young (18–39 years) people with type 1 or type 2 diabetes and metabolic syndrome. Indeed, statin and aspirin treatment should be considered in most patients with metabolic syndrome, as the majority of these patients will have CVD risk of over 20%.

Further reading

Adler AI, Stratton IM, Neil HA, *et al.* Association of systolic blood pressure with macrovascular and microvascular complications of type 2 diabetes (UKPDS 36): prospective observational study. *BMJ* 2000; **321**: 412–19.

Alberti KGMM, Zimmet P, Shaw J for the IDF Epidemiology Task Force Consensus Group. The metabolic syndrome – a new worldwide definition. *Lancet* 2005; **366**: 1059–62.

Chung NAY, Lip GYH, Beevers DG. Hypertension in old age. *CPD Journal Intern Med* 2001; **2**: 46–9.

Cohn JN, Tognoni G. A randomized trial of the angiotensin-receptor blocker valsartan in chronic heart failure. *N Engl J Med* 2001; **345**: 1667–75.

Edmunds E, Lip GY. Cardiovascular risk in women: the cardiologist's perspective. *QJM* 2000; **93**: 135–45.

Felmeden DC, Lip GY, Beevers G. Calcium antagonists in

diabetic hypertension. *Diabetes Obes Metab* 2001; **3**: 311–18.

Gibbs CR, Beevers DG, Lip GY. The management of hypertensive disease in black patients. *QJM* 1999; **92**: 187–92.

Grundy SM, Brewer B, Cleeman JI, *et al*. Definition of metabolic syndrome. Report of the National Heart, Lung and Blood Institute/American Heart Association Conference on scientific issues related to definition. *Circulation* 2004; **109**: 433–8.

Lip GY, Beevers M, Beevers DG, Dillon MJ. The measurement of blood pressure and the detection of hypertension in children and adolescents. *J Hum Hypertens* 2001; **15**: 419–23.

PROGRESS Collaborative Group. Randomised trial of a perindopril-based blood-pressure-lowering regimen among 6,105 individuals with previous stroke or transient ischaemic attack. *Lancet* 2001; **358**: 1033–41.

Stratton IM, Adler AI, Neil HA, *et al*. Association of glycaemia with macrovascular and microvascular complications of type 2 diabetes (UKPDS 35): prospective observational study. *BMJ* 2000; **321**: 405–12.

UK Prospective Diabetes Study (UKPDS) Group. Cost effectiveness analysis of improved blood pressure control in hypertensive patients with type 2 diabetes: UKPDS 40. *BMJ* 1998; **317**: 720–6.

UK Prospective Diabetes Study Group. Efficacy of atenolol and captopril in reducing risk of macrovascular and microvascular complications in type 2 diabetes: UKPDS 39. *BMJ* 1998; **317**: 713–20.

UK Prospective Diabetes Study Group. Tight blood pressure control and risk of macrovascular and microvascular complications in type 2 diabetes: UKPDS 38. *BMJ* 1998; **317**: 703–13.

UK Prospective Diabetes Study Group. Intensive blood-glucose control with sulphonylureas or insulin compared with conventional treatment and risk of complications in patients with type 2 diabetes (UKPDS 33). *Lancet* 1998; **352**: 837–53.

Vora JP, Ibrahim HA, Bakris GL. Responding to the challenge of diabetic nephropathy: the historic evolution of detection, prevention and management. *J Hum Hypertens* 2000; **14**: 667–85.

Yusuf S, Sleight P, Pogue J, *et al*. Effects of an angiotensin-converting-enzyme inhibitor, ramipril on cardiovascular events in high-risk patients. Heart Outcomes Prevention Evaluation Study Investigators. *N Engl J Med* 2000; **342**: 145–53.

8. Hypertension in pregnancy

Classification of hypertension in pregnancy
Pre-existing essential hypertension
Secondary hypertension in pregnancy
Pregnancy-induced hypertension
Pre-eclampsia
Eclampsia
Choice of antihypertensive therapy in pregnancy
Treatment of pre-eclampsia and eclampsia
Further pregnancy

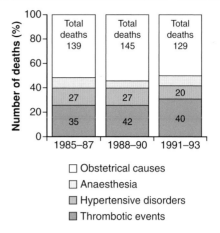

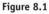

□ Obstetrical causes
□ Anaesthesia
▨ Hypertensive disorders
▦ Thrombotic events

Figure 8.1
Causes of maternal deaths in the UK from 1985 to 1993.

The management of hypertension in pregnancy is a specialist area and a detailed treatise is beyond the scope of this book. Hypertension occurs in around 5% of all pregnancies. However, this covers a wide range of conditions that carry different implications for pregnancy outcome and require different management strategies. Raised blood pressure (BP) may also be a marker of underlying maternal disease or it may be a consequence of pregnancy itself. It is important to remember that hypertension in pregnancy affects the fetus as well as the mother. It can result in fetal growth retardation and, if severe, both maternal and fetal morbidity and mortality (Figure 8.1). If recognized early and managed appropriately, many of these complications can be reduced. Hypertension may be the first sign of impending pre-eclampsia – a potentially more serious condition of the second half of pregnancy and the puerperium. When measuring BP in pregnant women, diastolic BP should be measured at the

disappearance of all sounds (phase V) and not at muffling (phase IV) as recommended in the past.

Hypertensive diseases in pregnancy, including pre-eclampsia, remain major causes of maternal and fetal mortality in the UK (the mortality rate is around 2%). Although maternal mortality due to hypertension has fallen markedly over the past three decades, eclampsia remains an important cause of a significant number of deaths. Eclampsia is responsible for one-sixth of all maternal deaths and a doubling of perinatal mortality. Despite accurate figures on the effects of raised BP, the precise causes of hypertension in pregnancy are unknown, and eclampsia has been referred to as the 'disease of theories'.

Classification of hypertension in pregnancy

There have been several attempts at classifying hypertension in pregnancy, although none is entirely satisfactory. This is partly because the diagnoses are often made in retrospect after the pregnancy is over. It is important to understand the different types of hypertension in pregnancy, not least because their prognosis differs widely. The current classification is based on the International Society for the Study of Hypertension in Pregnancy (ISSHP) recommendations (Table 8.1). In 1997, Brown and Buddle published a comparison of the criteria of the Australasian Society for the Study of Hypertension in Pregnancy and the International Society for the Study of Hypertension in 17,657 consecutive pregnancies, of which 1183 (6.7%) were complicated by hypertension (Figure 8.2).

In this above classification the term 'pregnancy-induced hypertension' is abolished. Some of these patients would have chronic hypertension while others have mild early pre-eclampsia (see Brown MA and Buddle ML. *J Hypertens* 1997; **15**: 1049–54).

Table 8.1
A simple classification of the hypertensive disorders of pregnancy

Raised blood pressure (>140/90 mmHg) before 20 weeks gestation
● Known chronic hypertension
  —essential
  —renal (glomerulonephritis, pyelonephritis, polycystic kidney disease)
  —renovascular (fibromuscular dysplasia)
  —adrenal (phaeochromocytoma)
● Presumed chronic hypertension

Raised blood pressure (>140/90 mmHg) after 20 weeks gestation
● Chronic hypertension
● Mild non-proteinuric pre-eclampsia
● Proteinuric pre-eclampsia
● Pre-eclampsia complicating chronic hypertension

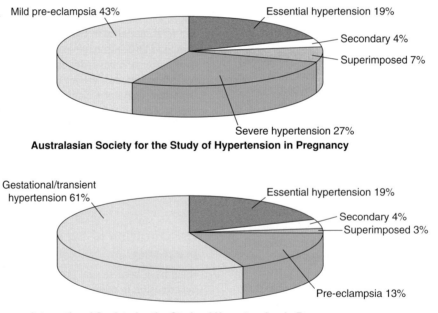

Mild pre-eclampsia 43% Essential hypertension 19%
Secondary 4%
Superimposed 7%
Severe hypertension 27%
Australasian Society for the Study of Hypertension in Pregnancy

Gestational/transient hypertension 61% Essential hypertension 19%
Secondary 4%
Superimposed 3%
Pre-eclampsia 13%

International Society for the Study of Hypertension in Pregnancy

Figure 8.2
Classifications of the hypertensive syndromes of pregnancy: the Australasian Society for the Study of Hypertension in Pregnancy classification and the International Society for the Study of Hypertension in Pregnancy classification. (Adapted from Brown et al. J Hypertens 1997; **15**: 1049–54.)

Pre-existing essential hypertension

This is otherwise referred to as chronic hypertension and is present before the 20th week of pregnancy. It is assumed the mother had pre-existing hypertension (although often no data are available). For this reason, chronic hypertension refers to long-term hypertension that is not confined to or caused by pregnancy, but may be revealed for the first time during pregnancy. About 5% of women of childbearing age have chronic pre-existing hypertension, which is usually mild. In women in their late 30s and 40s, this figure approaches 10%. Mild essential hypertension in pregnancy does not appear to carry a bad prognosis for the mother or fetus and its early treatment does not convincingly prevent the onset of pre-eclampsia. The condition is defined by the World Health Organization criteria as BP >140/90 mmHg.

The usual 'cause' of chronic hypertension is essential hypertension. However, there may be other infrequent secondary causes.

> Chronic hypertension is long-term hypertension that is first discovered during the first 20 weeks of pregnancy, but is not caused by the pregnancy

Secondary hypertension in pregnancy

This is uncommon, but is accounted for by causes of secondary hypertension in younger people, such as phaeochromocytoma, renal disease and primary hyperaldosteronism. For example, phaeochromocytoma is well-described in association with pregnancy and is associated with a poor maternal and fetal outcome. Hypertension associated with renal disease may exacerbate renal impairment, resulting in poor outcome of the pregnancy, deterioration of renal function across pregnancy and subsequent subfertility.

Pregnancy-induced hypertension

Pregnancy-induced hypertension usually develops after the 20th week of pregnancy and usually resolves 10 days after delivery. For this diagnosis to be made, BP must be documented to be normal both before and after pregnancy. Therefore, this diagnosis may sometimes only be made retrospectively.

The definitions of pregnancy-induced hypertension vary. The ISSHP defines pregnancy-induced hypertension as a single diastolic (phase V) BP >110 mmHg or two readings of >90 mmHg at least four hours apart, occurring after the 20th week of pregnancy. The US National High Blood Pressure Education Program defines it as a rise of >15 mmHg diastolic or 30 mmHg systolic compared to readings taken in early pregnancy.

A concise clinical definition by Davey and MacGillivray describes the condition as 'the occurrence of a BP of 140/90 mmHg or more on at least two separate occasions a minimum of six hours apart in a woman known to have been normotensive before this time, and in whom the BP has returned to normal limits by the sixth postpartum week'.

The threshold at which drug treatment is recommended is emphatically not 140/90 mmHg. Many young pregnant women may in fact show the BP increase required for the diagnosis of pre-eclampsia without increasing their pressure to 140/90 mmHg. Pregnancy-induced hypertension affects up to 25% of women in their first pregnancy and in 10% of subsequent pregnancies.

> Pregnancy-induced hypertension can be defined as a BP of ≥ 140/90 mmHg measured on at least two separate occasions at least six hours apart, when the patient had been normotensive before pregnancy

If pregnancy-induced hypertension is mild and does not progress to pre-eclampsia or eclampsia, the prognosis is usually good. However, women who develop hypertension early in the second half of pregnancy are more likely to progress to pre-eclampsia. They may develop proteinuria, thrombocytopenia, oedema and may need an early delivery.

Pre-eclampsia

Pregnancy-induced hypertension (BP >140/90 mmHg) after the 20th week of pregnancy that is associated with proteinuria (>300 mg/L), is often referred to as pre-eclampsia. This commonly occurs in primigravidae in the second half of pregnancy and marks a severe, acute change in the mother's condition. Although pre-eclampsia is defined as presenting after 20 weeks, it may often occur earlier or become evident only after delivery. The incidence of proteinuric pre-eclampsia is approximately 1 in 20–30 pregnancies in the UK.

Risk factors for pre-eclampsia

The risk factors for pre-eclampsia include fetal-specific and maternal-specific factors, discussed in detail below (Table 8.2). For example, pre-eclampsia is more common in primigravidae, those aged under 20 years or over 35 years, or in women with previous severe pre-eclampsia. It is thought there is also a genetic predisposition to pre-eclampsia.

Pre-eclampsia is also more common in women who are overweight and of short stature, and in women with chronic hypertension, especially those with associated chronic renal disease. Women with chronic hypertension are three to seven times more likely to develop higher BP and proteinuria (often referred to as 'superimposed pre-eclampsia') than normotensive women.

The patient is usually (not always) symptomatic with frontal headaches and visual symptoms (jagged, angular flashes at the periphery of her visual fields, loss of vision in some areas) due to cerebral oedema. There is often epigastric pain due to hepatic oedema and occasionally an itch over the mask region of the face.

Table 8.2
Pathogenesis of pre-eclampsia – failure of the normal demuscularization of the uterine spiral arteries in early pregnancy

- Predisposing factors:
  —prior hypertension
  —prior diabetes mellitus
  —increased insulin resistance
  —increased testosterone
  —increased triglycerides, decreased HDL and increased small dense LDL cholesterol
  —African origin
  —first pregnancy
  —changed paternity
  —multiple pregnancy
  —hydatidiform mole
  —fetal chromosomal abnormalities
  —placental hydrops
- Pathophysiological and clinical aspects:
  —raised blood pressure
  —proteinuria
  —reduced multi-organ perfusion
  —reduced uterine blood flow
  —increased sensitivity to pressor agents
  —vasospasm
  —reduced plasma volume
  —increased extravascular fluid volume
  —activation of coagulation cascade
  —platelet activation
  —microthrombi formation

> Short, overweight women and women with chronic hypertension are most susceptible to pre-eclampsia

Clinical signs

On examination, BP may be high and there is a sharp increase in proteinuria. Hypertension usually precedes proteinuria but the converse is occasionally encountered. Blood pressures are usually unstable at rest, and circadian rhythm is altered, initially with a loss of physiological nocturnal dipping; in severe cases there is 'reverse dipping' with the highest BP seen at night.

Early papilloedema may be seen on fundoscopy. There may be increased and brisk reflexes and clonus. Oedema is a less reliable diagnostic feature as mild pre-tibial and facial oedema are commonly found in normal pregnancy. Urgent antihypertensive and anticonvulsant treatment is needed. It should be noted that pregnancy-induced hypertension with or without proteinuria may be superimposed on chronic hypertension.

Eclampsia

Eclampsia is a hypertensive emergency associated with a high incidence of both maternal and fetal death. This is a convulsive condition usually associated with proteinuric pregnancy-induced hypertension, occurring in around one in 500 pregnancies.

Clinical signs

The condition resembles other forms of hypertensive encephalopathy, with similar symptoms of headache, nausea, vomiting and convulsions. BP is invariably high and proteinuria >300 mg/L is almost always present. There may be gross oedema and convulsions – if they occur, they usually develop in labour or in the puerperium. Auras, epigastric pain, apprehension and hyperreflexia may precede the convulsions, with little or no warning in many cases.

After intense tonic-clonic seizures, the patient may become stuporose or comatose. Another complication common to eclampsia and hypertensive encephalopathy is cortical blindness, which results from petechial haemorrhages and focal oedema in the occipital cortex. Other complications include pulmonary oedema, renal failure, hepatic failure, retinal detachment and cerebrovascular accidents.

Choice of antihypertensive therapy in pregnancy

Methyldopa remains the antihypertensive drug of choice for idiopathic hypertension or pre-eclampsia because of its long and extensive use without reports of serious adverse effects on the fetus. As a centrally acting anti-

hypertensive agent, methyldopa may be associated with depression and sedation. Autoimmune haemolytic anaemia is also recognized with methyldopa, which necessitates discontinuation of therapy.

Calcium antagonists (especially slow-release nifedipine) and the vasodilator hydralazine are common second-line drugs. Sublingual nifedipine should never be used. Both of these vasodilators may be associated with reflex tachycardia and may work synergistically with beta-blockers. Side-effects are uncommon with short-term use of hydralazine.

Labetalol (alpha-blocker and beta-blocker) is also widely used as a second-line agent, particularly for resistant hypertension in the third trimester. However, ACE inhibitors and angiotensin II antagonists are contraindicated in pregnancy due to adverse effects on the fetus. Beta-blockers such as atenolol may result in small babies (Figure 8.3).

Contraindicated drug therapy

Before 28 weeks' gestation, beta-blockers are not widely used because of concerns that they may inhibit fetal growth. The diuretics may

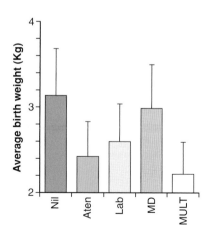

Figure 8.3
Antihypertensive drugs and fetal growth. Aten, atenolol; Lab, labetalol; MD, methyldopa; MULT, multiple drugs. (Adapted from Lydakis *et al. Am J Hypertens* 1999; **12**: 541–7.)

reduce the incidence of pre-eclampsia, although no benefit was shown on fetal outcome. In theory at least, they may reduce the already decreased circulatory blood volume in women with pre-eclampsia and compromise utero–placental circulation.

ACE inhibitors and angiotensin II receptor antagonists should be avoided because they may cause oligohydramnios, renal failure, hypotension and intrauterine death in the fetus. Hypertensive women who are planning a pregnancy or who become pregnant while on antihypertensive treatment should be advised to change their therapy to one of the drugs recommended as safe for the treatment of hypertension in pregnancy (Table 8.3).

Use of prophylactic aspirin

The Australasian Society for the Study of Hypertension in Pregnancy (ASSHP) recommends use of prophylactic low-dose aspirin from early pregnancy in the following groups:

- women with prior fetal loss after the first trimester due to placental insufficiency
- women with severe fetal growth retardation in a preceding pregnancy either due to pre-eclampsia or unexplained causes

Table 8.3
Drug treatments for hypertension in pregnancy

- Contraindicated
  —ACE inhibitors
  —calcium channel blockers in mild hypertension
  —thiazides
  —atenolol, propranolol
- Probably safe
  —methyldopa, particularly in asthmatic mothers
  —alpha-blockers
  —some beta-blockers, e.g. labetalol, oxprenolol, pindolol
  —nifedipine in severe cases
- Emergency
  —intravenous and intramuscular drugs, e.g. hydralazine, labetalol
  —anticonvulsants
  —magnesium sulphate

- women with severe early-onset pre-eclampsia in a previous pregnancy requiring delivery at or before 32 weeks gestation.

Aspirin is not indicated routinely for healthy nulliparous women, women with mild chronic hypertension and women with established pre-eclampsia.

Treatment of pre-eclampsia and eclampsia

Urgent transfer to a specialized maternity unit with an adequate special care baby unit is indicated together with antihypertensive and anticonvulsant therapy. Diazepam and magnesium sulphate prevent fits and reduce BP.

The first line of management is to control the seizures. If at home, the woman should be laid on her side and an airway established. Intravenous diazepam, usually 20–40 mg, is used. Intravenous magnesium sulphate has been shown to improve outcome in eclampsia and is regarded as first-line treatment as an anticonvulsant in eclampsia. Intravenous magnesium also has antihypertensive properties. Occasionally phenytoin is used to prevent recurrence of fits.

Intravenous hydralazine is widely used as an antihypertensive drug of first choice, given as a 5 mg bolus at 20 minutes or as an infusion of 25 mg in 500 ml of Hartman's solution. The dose is titrated against the BP. An alternative is an intravenous infusion of labetalol. If the woman is in labour or induction is considered, an epidural anaesthetic may be helpful both to lower the BP and to reduce the tendency to fit by reducing the pain of uterine contractions. The ultimate treatment of eclampsia is, however, urgent delivery of the baby.

Magnesium sulphate is the first-line drug to treat eclampsia seizures

Further pregnancy

Mothers who have had pre-eclampsia during a first pregnancy should be warned of a 7.5% risk that it might return for their second. A history of spontaneous or induced first trimester abortion in a first pregnancy does not confer the same relative immunity to severe pre-eclampsia in the subsequent pregnancy. Other causes of hypertension should be considered when a patient develops hypertension in pregnancy, especially if there are any unusual features or the hypertension is severe.

Women with previous pre-eclampsia who become pregnant again should be targeted for management in a joint antenatal and BP clinic. Such women are also usually regarded as being more likely to develop essential hypertension in later life and regular screening for hypertension is recommended (Table 8.4). If a woman with a history of hypertension in pregnancy wishes oral contraception (this is not a contraindication), careful BP monitoring is essential. The developmental status of children born to women with pre-eclampsia is usually good.

> Women who develop pre-eclampsia during their first pregnancy have a 7.5% risk of it returning for their next pregnancy, and should be monitored at joint antenatal and BP clinics

The benefits of treating hypertension in pregnancy are summed up in Table 8.5. Clearly the best data are for the treatment of pre-eclampsia/eclampsia, with benefits for both the mother and baby, especially in the presence of severe hypertension. These uncertainties over the benefits of treatment are compounded by a recent meta-analysis suggesting that over-aggressive BP reduction in pregnancy is associated with a greater odds ratio for small-for-gestational-age babies and lower birth weights.

In a paper by von Dadelszen *et al.* (2000), the relation between fetoplacental growth and the use of oral antihypertensive medication to treat

Table 8.4
Laboratory tests used for hypertension in pregnancy

Test	Rationale
Full blood count	Haemoconcentration is found in pre-eclampsia and is an indicator of severity Decreased platelet count suggests severe pre-eclampsia
Blood film	Signs of microangiopathic haemolytic anaemia favour the diagnosis of pre-eclampsia
Urinalysis	If dipstick proteinuria of +1 or more, a quantitative measurement of 24-hour protein excretion is required Hypertensive pregnant women with proteinuria should be considered to have pre-eclampsia until proven otherwise
Biochemistry, including serum creatinine, urate and liver function tests	Abnormal or rising levels suggest pre-eclampsia and are an indicator of disease severity
Lactate dehydrogenase	Elevated levels are associated with haemolysis and hepatic involvement, suggesting severe pre-eclampsia
Serum albumin	Levels may be decreased even with mild proteinuria, perhaps owing to capillary leak or hepatic involvement in pre-eclampsia

(Adapted from recommendations of the National High Blood Pressure Education Program Working Group Report on High Blood Pressure in Pregnancy. *Am J Obstet Gynecol* 1990; **163**: 1689–712.)

mild-to-moderate pregnancy hypertension was assessed using a metaregression analysis of published data from randomized controlled trials. The change in (group) mean arterial pressure (MAP) from enrolment to delivery was compared with indicators of fetoplacental growth. They found that greater mean difference in MAP with antihypertensive therapy was associated with the

Table 8.5 (a)

Are there benefits of treating hypertension during pregnancy?

	Mother	Fetus
Pre-existing hypertension	Yes	No
Pregnancy-induced hypertension	No	No
Pre-eclampsia	Yes	Yes

Table 8.5 (b)

Antihypertensive therapy for chronic hypertension during pregnancy

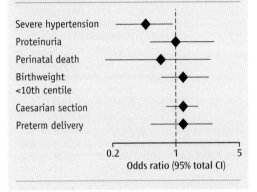

birth of a higher proportion of small-for-gestational-age (SGA) infants (slope: 0.09 [SD 0.03], r^2=0.48, P=0.006, 14 trials) and lower mean birthweight significant after exclusion of data from another paper regarded as an extreme statistical outliner (slope: −14.49 [6.98] r^2=0.16, P=0.049, 27 trials). No relation with mean placental weight was seen (slope −2.01 [1.62], r^2=0.15, P=0.25, 11 trials). This analysis

therefore suggests that treatment-induced falls in maternal blood pressure may adversely affect fetal growth. As discussed above, in view of the small maternal benefits that are likely to be derived from therapy, more information on relative maternal and fetal benefits and risks of oral antihypertensive drug treatment of *mild-to-moderate* pregnancy hypertension may be required.

Further reading

Broughton Pipkin F, Roberts JM. Hypertension in pregnancy. *J Hum Hypertens* 2000; **14**: 705–24.

Brown MA, Buddle ML. What's in a name? Problems with the classification of hypertension in pregnancy. *J Hypertens* 1997; **15**: 1049–54.

Chung NAY, Beevers DG, Lip GYH. Management of hypertension in pregnancy. *Am J Cardiovasc Drugs* 2001; **1**: 253–62.

Dekker G, Sibai B. Primary, secondary, and tertiary prevention of pre-eclampsia. *Lancet* 2001; **357**: 209–15.

Department of Health and Social Security. Report on confidential enquiries into maternal deaths in England and Wales 1982–84. London: HMSO, 1986: 10–19.

Ferrer RL, Sibai BM, Mulrow CD, *et al.* Management of mild chronic hypertension during pregnancy: a review. *Obstet Gynecol* 2000; **96**: 849–60.

Granger JP, Alexander BT, Bennett WA, *et al.* Pathophysiology of pregnancy-induced hypertension. *Am J Hypertens* 2001; **14**: 178S–85S.

Lydakis C, Lip GY, Beevers M, *et al.* Atenolol and fetal growth in pregnancies complicated by hypertension. *Am J Hypertens* 1999; **12**: 541–7.

Sibai BM. Antihypertensive drugs during pregnancy. *Semin Perinatol* 2001; **25**: 159–64.

von Dadelszen P, Ornstein MP, Bull SB, *et al.* Fall in mean arterial pressure and fetal growth restriction in pregnancy hypertension: a meta-analysis. *Lancet* 2000; **355**: 87–92.

9. Hypertensive urgencies and emergencies

Epidemiology
Malignant hypertension
Pathophysiology
Clinical features
Physical signs
Early management
Summary

Table 9.1
Hypertensive crises

- Hypertensive emergencies
  —hypertensive encephalopathy
  —hypertensive left ventricular failure
  —hypertension with myocardial infarction or unstable angina
  —hypertension with aortic dissection
  —severe hypertension with subarachnoid haemorrhage or stroke
  —acute renal failure
  —phaeochromocytoma crisis
  —recreational drugs (amphetamines, LSD, cocaine, ecstasy)
  —microangiopathic haemolytic anaemia
  —perioperative hypertension*

*This should be given individual consideration given the unique clinical factors present during the perioperative period

A number of different terms have been applied to severe elevations of blood pressure (BP) (>180/110 mmHg). In general, 'hypertensive emergencies' are defined as severe elevations in blood pressure with associated end-organ damage of the central nervous system (CNS), the cardiovascular system and the kidneys. The term 'hypertensive urgencies' is used for patients with severely elevated BP without evidence of acute end-organ damage. Hypertensive encephalopathy, hypertensive left ventricular failure and acute aortic dissection are immediately life-threatening and are considered to be true hypertensive emergencies (Table 9.1). The term 'malignant hypertension' is defined as a syndrome of elevated BP accompanied by encephalopathy or nephropathy.

It is important to have coherent strategies for the diagnosis, investigation and management of hypertensive crises, as the mortality in these patients is high and rapid treatment of hypertension may itself be hazardous. These risks are greatly increased when patients are treated with inappropriate pharmacological agents in the absence of appropriate monitoring.

Epidemiology

There has been a decline in the prevalence of hypertensive crises over the past 20 years, probably as a result of more effective diagnosis and treatment of milder grades of hypertension. Hypertension crises are now reported to be rare in western developed populations, although still reported to be common in some developing countries.

Nevertheless, in Birmingham (UK), the incidence of hypertensive crises does not appear to have fallen substantially over the past 25 years, with an estimated annual incidence of 1–2 per 100,000 population (Figure 9.1). The incidence of hypertensive crises is higher in the Afro-Caribbean population and the elderly. The majority of patients have a history of hypertension and many would have been prescribed antihypertensive therapy with inadequate BP control.

Malignant hypertension

Hypertensive crises may present at any age, including the elderly, and recurrent clinical presentations of malignant-phase hypertension may occur. Severe hypertension in young women

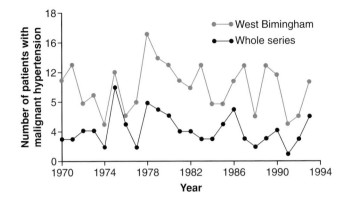

Figure 9.1
Failure of malignant hypertension to decline in Birmingham, UK.

has been related to both the use of the oral contraceptive pill and a history of hypertension in pregnancy. Several studies have also reported an association between cigarette smoking and malignant hypertension.

Demographic and socioeconomic factors appear to be important and may contribute to the failure of malignant hypertension cases to decline in some areas of the world. Malignant hypertension is reported to occur more frequently in patients from lower socioeconomic groups and in subjects with high self-perceived 'stress' levels. Ethnicity may be important, as closer examination of the Birmingham cohort reveals a high prevalence in first-generation migrant groups, including Afro-Caribbeans (mainly from Jamaica) and Asians (mainly from Punjabi-speaking areas of India and Pakistan). In this respect, the Birmingham cohort resembles other series of malignant hypertensive patients from less developed countries (for example, South Africa).

A further reason for the failure of malignant hypertension to decline might be the presence of patients who have limited understanding of the nature and complications of the disease, and the importance of compliance with antihypertensive treatment.

> Hypertensive crises may be found in any age group, including the elderly, and studies have linked them to demographic and ethnic factors

Causes of malignant hypertension

Hypertensive crises are more likely to be associated with an underlying cause (Table 9.2). Conn's syndrome (primary hyperaldosteronism) is reported to be rare in cases of malignant hypertension.

Prognosis

In the modern era, the more effective management of hypertension has led to an improvement in five-year survival rates, in developed countries, from 60% to 75% (Figure 9.2). Nevertheless, in developing countries such as Nigeria, the prognosis continues to be poor with only 40% of patients surviving longer than one year.

Early recognition

Early recognition of malignant hypertension is important as patients tend to develop overt clinical symptoms at a late stage of the disease. In the long term, the most common causes of death in patients with a history of malignant hypertension are chronic renal failure (40%),

Table 9.2
Underlying causes in studies of patients with malignant hypertension

	Glasgow	Leicester	Johannesburg	Birmingham
Follow-up	1968–83	1974–83	1979–80	1970–93
Number of patients	139	100	62	242
Underlying causes (%)				
—essential	60	68	82	56
—renal	18	19	5	28
—renovascular	14	6	3	2
—other	8	7	10	10

cerebrovascular disease (24%), myocardial infarction (11%) and heart failure (10%).

Cigarette smoking exerts an adverse effect on prognosis in patients who continue to smoke following their initial presentation.

Renal function continues to deteriorate in some patients with malignant hypertension despite good BP control during follow-up. Nevertheless, the quality of the BP control does predict the long-term prognosis and BP should be optimized with the target BP of 125/75 mmHg.

> The most common causes of death in patients with a history of malignant hypertension are chronic renal failure, cerebrovascular disease, myocardial infarction and heart failure

Pathophysiology

Malignant hypertension is characterized by fibrinoid necrosis of arterioles in many sites, including the kidneys, eyes, brain, heart and gut. However, this histological feature is not pathognomonic of malignant hypertension. Subintimal cellular proliferation of the interlobular arteries of the kidney is also commonly seen and this may well be important as intimal thickening may lead to luminal occlusion in these small vessels. The occlusion of these small arteries contributes to chronic renal ischaemia, leading to the renal failure that is often seen in malignant hypertension.

Microscopic examination of the arterioles reveals alternating bands of constriction and dilation. These dilated segments are thought to represent focal areas of disruption of the vessel wall related to the rapid rise in intraluminal pressure, and these areas have been shown to be abnormally permeable to plasma proteins. Such disruption of the vessel wall leads to the deposition of fibrin, and therefore fibrinoid necrosis. This process may lead to the further deposition of fibrin in the vessel wall and microcirculation, as well as platelet

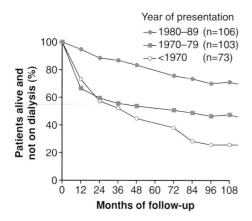

Figure 9.2
Survival of malignant hypertension. (Adapted from Lip *et al.* *J Hypertens* 1995; **13**: 915.)

aggregation, release of growth factors, subintimal cellular proliferation and activation of the coagulation system, which may result in microangiopathic haemolytic anaemia – a recognized feature in some of these patients. In addition, ischaemia of the juxtaglomerular apparatus leads to activation of the renin–angiotensin system with further vasoconstriction and arteriolar damage.

> Malignant hypertension is marked by fibrinoid necrosis of arterioles in sites such as the kidneys, eyes, brain, heart and gut

Cerebral and renal autoregulation

Blood flow and perfusion of the brain and kidneys are maintained over a range of blood pressures – so-called autoregulation. In healthy humans, this autoregulatory mechanism maintains normal cerebral blood flow between a systemic arterial blood pressure of 60 mmHg to 120 mmHg. With chronic hypertension, the pressure-flow autoregulation curve is shifted to the right such that cerebral blood flow is maintained at a higher range of blood pressure.

While this adaptation to chronic hypertension protects the brain and kidneys from chronically elevated BP, a sudden drop in BP (even to 'normal' levels) may result in reduced blood flow to these organs. Cerebral autoregulation is also impaired at extremely high BP levels and in hypertensive encephalopathy, making cerebral perfusion exquisitely sensitive to changes in systemic blood pressure changes. Clearly, these autoregulatory mechanisms have important implications for the practical management of hypertensive emergencies (see below).

Clinical features

Severe hypertension may be an incidental finding in an asymptomatic patient, although associated symptoms may be present. The presenting symptoms of malignant hypertension are variable, although headaches and visual

disturbances are the most common. Initial symptoms are often non-specific and include anorexia, nausea, vomiting and abdominal pain. These non-specific symptoms often lead to delayed diagnosis and treatment. Breathlessness due to left ventricular failure might be present but ischaemic chest pain is less common.

Aortic dissection must be considered in any patient who presents with raised BP and severe pain in the back, chest or abdomen.

Hypertensive encephalopathy is rare and usually occurs in patients with a history of hypertension that has been inadequately treated, or where previous treatment has been discontinued. It may be associated with severe headache, nausea, vomiting, visual disturbances and confusion may also be a feature. However, with the advent of high-resolution CT scanning it has become clear that many patients who are thought to have hypertensive encephalopathy, have actually suffered an acute stroke.

> The most common symptoms of malignant hypertension are headaches and visual disturbances, with non-specific initial symptoms including anorexia, nausea, vomiting and abdominal pain

Physical signs
Retinopathy

Malignant hypertension is confirmed by the presence of advanced retinal hypertensive changes. Clinical decisions, in patients with severe hypertension, should be based on the presence or absence of retinopathy together with the height of the BP.

The Keith, Wagener and Barker classification (see Table 4.7), originally proposed in 1939, remains the most commonly used grading system for hypertensive retinopathy. The strength of this classification is the correlation between the clinical signs and prognosis, although this grading system has a number of limitations. In particular, there is no significant difference in the long-term prognosis between grades III and IV hypertensive retinopathy.

The restrictions of this traditional classification for hypertensive retinopathy have led to the development of a simplified grading system, which is more applicable to modern clinical practice (Table 9.3). In this grading system, arteriolar narrowing and focal constriction, features which correlate with BP levels, age and general cardiovascular status, constitute the first grade (grade I). The presence of retinal haemorrhages or exudates, cotton wool spots (with or without papilloedema) constitute the second and prognostically more significant grade (grade II) (Figure 9.3).

An additional subgroup of patients has been identified who have isolated bilateral papilloedema, in association with severe hypertension (Figure 9.4). The clinical

Table 9.3
Revised grading system for hypertensive retinopathy

Grade	Retinal changes	Hypertensive category	Prognosis
I 'Non-malignant'	Generalized arteriolar narrowing Focal constriction (NB not arteriovenous nipping)	Established hypertension	May depend on height of blood pressure, but age and other concomitant cardiovascular risk factors are equally important
II 'Malignant'	Haemorrhages, hard exudates, cotton wool spots ± Optic disc swelling	Accelerated or malignant hypertension with retinovascular damage present*	Most die within two years if untreated In treated patients, median survival is now >12 years

*To fulfil criteria of Grade II, retinovascular damage should be present in both eyes. Note that if carotid occlusive disease is present, ocular blood flow may be reduced and if asymmetrical this may be sufficient to mask papilloedema or other hypertensive changes in the ipsilateral eye.

(After Dodson *et al.* Hypertensive retinopathy: a review of existing classification systems and a suggestion for a simplified grading system. *J Human Hypertens* 1996; **10**: 93–8.)

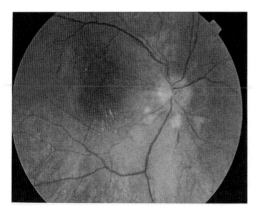 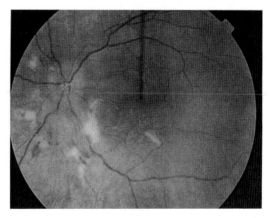

Figure 9.3
Malignant phase hypertension – retinal flame-shaped haemorrhages, cotton wool spots, exudates and papilloedema are visible.

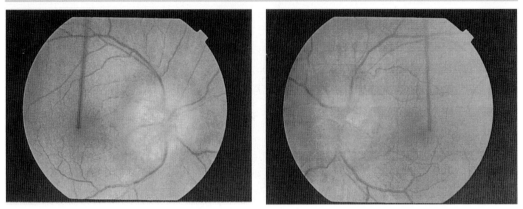

Figure 9.4
Lone papilloedema in a patient with severe hypertension, showing bilateral optic disc swelling and no other significant retinal features.

characteristics of these patients are similar to those with 'conventional' malignant hypertension, although they have been reported to have a shorter median survival. However, care is needed to differentiate such patients from those with benign intracranial hypertension, who are typically young, overweight and female. A CT scan and lumbar puncture may be needed to ascertain the diagnosis.

Other clinical signs

In addition to the retinopathy there may be signs of left heart failure, left ventricular hypertrophy and sometimes anaemia due to associated renal failure. Asymmetrical BP readings, absent pulses, aortic incompetence and neurological signs should raise the suspicion of acute aortic dissection. Fluctuating neurological signs, disorientation, reduced level of consciousness, neurological deficit and focal or generalized seizures are all potential manifestations of hypertensive encephalopathy. Severe injury to the kidneys may result in renal failure with oliguria, proteinuria and even haematuria.

Early management
As previously discussed, patients with chronic hypertension have rightward shifts in their

pressure-flow autoregulation curve. In addition, patients with severe malignant hypertension may have abnormal autoregulatory mechanisms. Consequently, over-rapid BP reductions are potentially hazardous and may lead to cerebral, renal or myocardial infarction, while visual loss is also a recognized complication of over-rapid treatment.

Any reduction in BP must be gradual and the approach to treatment governed by the presence (and type) or absence of end-organ damage, i.e. hypertensive emergency or urgency. Parenteral antihypertensive therapy is indicated in hypertensive emergencies, with the aim of lowering diastolic BP by about 15% to 110 mmHg over about 30–60 minutes (with the exception of aortic dissection). Blood pressure should not be lowered to 'normal' levels. Parenteral antihypertensive treatment is not indicated in hypertensive urgencies (without end-organ damage).

In general, parenteral therapy requires high-dependency monitoring and should be restricted to severe emergencies where complications such as hypertensive encephalopathy, left ventricular failure and aortic dissection are present. The choice of parenteral antihypertensive therapy is dependent on the type of end-organ damage.

Hypertensive encephalopathy

Sodium nitroprusside

Sodium nitroprusside is the drug of choice when neurological damage is thought to be imminent. It is a potentially dangerous drug and should only be administered in a high dependency unit with cardiac and BP monitoring.

Nitroprusside is administered as a continuous titrated infusion, which is increased to achieve a diastolic BP of 90–110 mmHg over 2–3 hours. Thiocyanate is the toxic metabolite of nitroprusside and its accumulation is more rapid in patients with renal and hepatic failure.

Labetalol

Parenteral labetalol has been successfully used in the treatment of hypertensive encephalopathy, although it has been reported to cause severe and unpredictable hypotension in some patients. Intravenous nitrates are of limited value in hypertensive encephalopathy because they cause headache at the doses required to bring about a substantial reduction in BP.

Arterial vasodilators

Diazoxide and hydralazine, both arterial vasodilators, were previously popular in the management of hypertensive crises. Diazoxide administered by rapid bolus injection has led to a number of cases of cerebral infarction and death, and it is now rarely indicated in the treatment of hypertensive crises. Hydralazine should also be avoided in hypertensive crises as the antihypertensive effects may be unpredictable, prolonged and not easily titrated.

Reflex tachycardia is associated with both diazoxide and hydralazine and these agents should be avoided in patients with known or suspected coronary disease.

In all cases of suspected hypertensive encephalopathy, if a reduction in BP is not accompanied by clinical improvement, then the diagnosis should be reconsidered.

Hypertensive left ventricular failure

Severe increases in systemic vascular resistance may result in left ventricular failure. In addition to the conventional management with opiates/opioids and loop diuretics, sodium nitroprusside is used to reduce pre-load and after-load. Nitrates may also be used, but are less potent.

Hypertension with unstable angina or myocardial infarction

In patients with severe hypertension and angina, intravenous nitrates are valuable as they reduce systemic vascular resistance and improve coronary perfusion. Beta-blockers, administered by slow intravenous injection (for example, 5 mg metoprolol repeated at intervals of 20 minutes) may be valuable when the BP is moderately raised, although in severe hypertension an intravenous infusion (for example, labetalol or esmolol) may be necessary. Sodium nitroprusside should be reserved for resistant cases, as it may exacerbate coronary ischaemia.

Aortic dissection

Effective blood pressure control is crucial in the management of aortic dissection. Indeed, prompt and effective BP control is the treatment of choice in type B aortic dissection (descending aorta distal to the subclavian artery). Propagation of the dissection is dependent not only on the elevation in BP but also the velocity of left ventricular ejection. Hence, specific therapy should be aimed at reducing BP and rate of pressure rise. Labetalol, with its beta-blocker effects, is the treatment of choice as it reduces the force of contraction, while sodium nitroprusside may be combined with a beta-blocker if further BP reduction is required. The aim of therapy should be to reduce the systolic BP to 100 mmHg in order to reduce aortic shear stress and limit the size of the dissection.

Stroke and subarachnoid haemorrhage

Cerebral autoregulation is commonly disturbed following an acute stroke. Excessive antihypertensive treatment may only serve to worsen the cerebral damage that results from an intracerebral infarction or haemorrhage. Antihypertensive treatment may lead to rapid and dangerous falls in BP, and should only be administered for severe elevations in BP (diastolic BP >130 mmHg). In these cases, oral therapy with small doses of slow-release nifedipine or atenolol may be indicated, although parenteral treatment is almost always contraindicated.

The calcium antagonist nimodipine has beneficial effects on cerebral vasospasm following subarachnoid haemorrhage, but these effects are not related to the small fall in BP.

Phaeochromocytoma

This condition is a rare cause of acute severe hypertension. The treatment of choice is the orally active short-acting alpha-blocker prazosin or phentolamine (which may also be given by bolus injection or infusion). It is possible to subsequently add a beta-blocker to control heart rate. Labetalol has also been used, while nitroprusside should be reserved for resistant cases.

Alpha-blockade is mandatory in the preoperative management of patients with phaeochromocytoma. It is used to overcome the intense vasoconstriction caused by the high circulating levels of adrenaline (epinephrine) and noradrenaline (norepinephrine).

Recreational drugs

Cocaine, ecstasy, amphetamines and LSD are among the sympathomimetic drugs that can produce severe acute hypertension. Isolated beta-blockade may lead to unopposed alpha-adrenergic effects, which may exacerbate the hypertensive crisis. Although labetalol has both alpha- and beta-blocking effects, controlled studies in animals and humans do not support its use. Nitroprusside, phentolamine or verapamil may be used.

Hypertensive urgencies

In the absence of acute end-organ damage, immediate BP reduction with parenteral drugs is not indicated. Indeed, this form of treatment may place the patient at unnecessary risk, as serious and sometimes fatal complications of treatment have been reported with almost all antihypertensive drugs (Table 9.4).

Table 9.4
Drug treatment in hypertensive crises

Drug	Administeration	Dose	Principal indications
Nifedipine	Oral	Start at 10 mg and repeat after 4–6 hours	Malignant hypertension
	Oral	Maintenance 10–40 mg twice daily	
Atenolol	Oral	Start at 25 mg Maximum 100 mg daily	Malignant hypertension
Sodium nitroprusside	i.v.	0.3–8 µg/kg/min Monitor levels in prolonged use	Hypertensive encephalopathy, left ventricular failure, dissecting aneurysm
Labetalol	i.v.	2 mg/min	Hypertensive encephalopathy, dissecting aneurysm, unstable angina or MI
Nitrates	i.v.	GTN 10–200 µg/min	Left ventricular failure, unstable angina with malignant hypertension

(GTN = glyceryl trinitrate; MI = myocardial infarction; i.v. = intravenous)

Oral therapy

An appropriate first-line oral agent is the slow-release nifedipine (10–20 mg in tablet form), which is a simple, effective and safe treatment and which does not significantly alter cerebral blood flow. Nifedipine capsules and sublingual nifedipine must not be used as their use has been reported to be associated with dramatic and unpredictable falls in BP, leading to cerebral and myocardial infarction.

Intensive care monitoring is not usually necessary. The dose of slow-release nifedipine may be repeated or increased at intervals of 6–12 hours, aiming for a gradual reduction in BP of 20–25% in the first 24 hours and to a diastolic BP of around 100 mmHg over the next few days.

> Slow-release nifedipine in tablet form is a first-line drug that does not alter cerebral blood flow significantly, but sublingual capsules must not be used

Angiotensin-converting enzyme (ACE) inhibitors

ACE inhibitors may produce rapid and dangerous falls in BP (particularly in patients with renovascular disease that might not be diagnosed in the acute situation) and are not recommended as first-line treatment. Diuretics should be restricted to those with evidence of fluid overload as patients with malignant hypertension are often volume depleted, secondary to pressure-related diuresis and activation of the renin–angiotensin system. In severe renal failure, haemodialysis or peritoneal dialysis may be indicated, particularly where there is gross fluid retention.

Combination treatment

Combination treatment is usually required in the long term. In the absence of contraindications, beta-blockers (e.g. atenolol) are an appropriate additional antihypertensive agent. It is sensible to start with small doses, such as atenolol 25 mg daily, increasing as necessary. The combination of atenolol and nifedipine is often a well-tolerated and effective regimen.

Summary

Although hypertensive crises are less common in modern-day medical practice, they are associated with significant morbidity and mortality rates as malignant hypertension remains a disease with a poor long-term prognosis.

In the majority of cases, rapid-onset orally active drugs are sufficient to control BP. Preparations of labetalol or sodium nitroprusside are occasionally necessary in cases of resistant hypertension and true hypertensive crises. However, clinicians should be aware of the hazards of the over-rapid reduction of BP in these patients as well as the complications of hypertension in the first place.

Further reading

Lim KG, Isles CG, Hodsman general practitioner, et al. Malignant hypertension in women of childbearing age and its relation to the contraceptive pill. Br Med J 1987; **294**: 1057–9.

Lip GYH, Beevers M, Beevers DG. The failure of malignant hypertension to decline: a survey of 24 years experience in a multiracial population in England. J Hypertens 1994; **12**: 1297–305.

Lip GYH, Beevers M, Beevers DG. Complications and survival of 315 patients with malignant hypertension. J Hypertens 1995; **13**: 915–24.

Lip GY, Beevers M, Beevers DG. Malignant hypertension in young women is related to previous hypertension in pregnancy not oral contraception. QJM 1997; **90**: 571–5.

Index